GYMNASTIC ACTIVITIES • DANCE • GAMES

PE LESSON PLANS

year 6

COMPLETE TEACHING PROGRAMME

SECOND EDITION

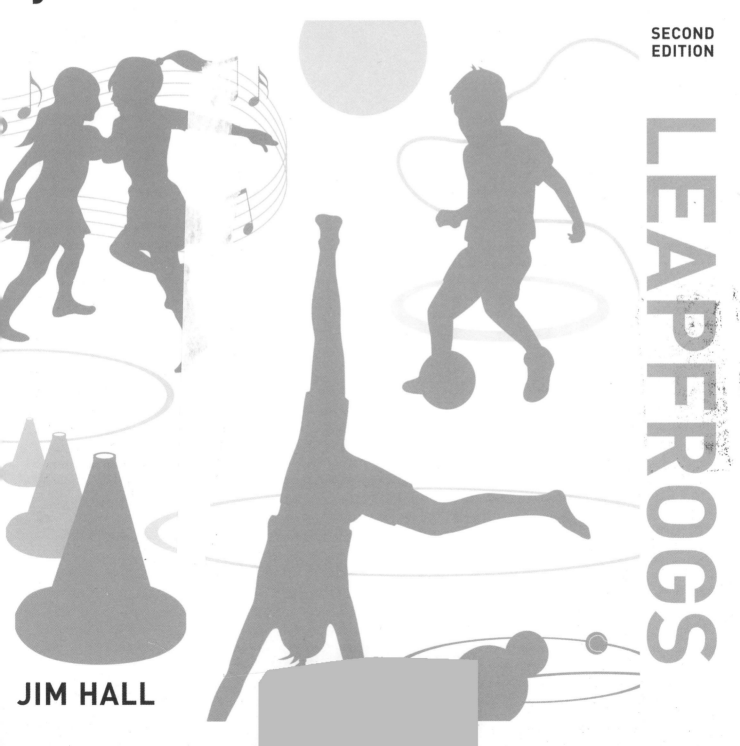

LEAPFROGS

JIM HALL

A music CD with tracks to accompany many of the Dance Lessons in this series is available separately (ISBN: 978 07136 7902 1)

Relevant tracks are indicated on each lesson page with the following logo:

Published in 2005 by A & C Black Publishers Ltd
36 Soho Square, London W1D 3QY
www.acblack.com

Second edition, 2009

ISBN 978 14081 0991 5

A CIP record for this book is available from the British Library.

Note: While every effort has been made to ensure that the content of this book is as technically accurate and as sound as possible, neither the author nor the publisher can accept responsibility for any injury or loss sustained as a result of the use of this material.

A & C Black uses paper produced with elemental chlorine-free pulp, harvested from managed sustainable forests.

Acknowledgements
Cover illustration by Tom Croft
Illustrations by Jan Smith
Cover design by James Watson

Typeset in 10pt DIN Regular.

Printed and bound in Great Britain b   Tweed.

Contents

Introduction

Because an increasing number of young children today do not have the opportunity to take part in regular play, physical activity or exercise, enjoyable, vigorous, well taught physical education lessons are more important than ever. Equally important is a sense of staff unity regarding the 'Why?', the 'What?', and the 'How?' of physical education to deliver a whole school, successful programme with continuity and high standards from year to year. The main reasons for teaching physical education, include:

Physical development. First and foremost, the main reason for teaching physical education has always been to inspire vigorous, enjoyable, challenging and wholehearted physical activity that develops normal healthy growth and satisfactory development of each pupil's strength, suppleness and stamina. The skills taught also aim to develop skilful, confident, well-controlled and safe movement. It is hoped that the varied skills will give pleasure and satisfaction, catering for many interests and aptitudes, and will eventually enable pupils to take part in healthy, worthwhile and sociable activities long after they have left school. These skills, learned and enjoyed at school, are remembered by the body for a very long time.

Personal, social and emotional development, compensating for the near total disappearance of play in the out-of-school lives of many of our pupils. It is reported that millions of children spend most of their free time – up to five hours every day – watching a TV or a computer screen. It has also been claimed that parents, who refuse to let their children go out to play, are producing a 'battery-farmed' generation who will never become resilient and will be unable to deal with risk.

This lack of play means no exercise, no fresh air, no physical development, no social development though interaction with others, no adventure in challenging situations and no emotional development. It has been said 'an individual's regard for, and attitude to, his or her physical self, especially at primary school age, is important to the development of self-image and the value given to self.' Physical education lessons are extremely visual, providing many opportunities for demonstrating success, creativity, versatility and enthusiastic performances which should be recognised by the teacher, praised and commented upon, and shared with others who should be encouraged to be warm in their praise and comments. Such successes can enhance a pupil's feelings of pride and self-confidence.

The play-like nature of physical education lessons is obvious. In games, running, jumping and landing, throwing and catching, batting, skipping, trying to score points or goals; in gymnastic activities, running, jumping and landing, rolling, climbing, swinging on ropes, balancing, circling on bars; and in dance, skipping, running and jumping, travelling with a partner, a group or a circle in performing a dance, are all playful actions in which pupils find fun and satisfaction from performing well, and social development from being in the company of others.

When teaching physical education lessons now, teachers need to remember that the lessons may be providing the only active play that some of the pupils will experience that week. The lessons must be vigorous, enjoyable, and give an impression of children at play.

Contributing to pupils' health now, and long after they have left school. The health of our children and eventually the health of our nation, has been a cause for concern for university researchers and health experts for decades. A 1997 headline described British children as 'The Flab Generation'. It was estimated in 2000, that in a class of thirty children, two will go on to have a heart attack, three will develop diabetes, and thirteen will become obese, all as result of a sedentary lifestyle and a diet dominated by chips, biscuits, sweets and sugary drinks. A 2002 report revealed that a third of 10 year olds did not even walk continuously for ten minutes a week.

The above statistics and figures have become far worse since those early ignored warnings. The NHS treated 85,000 patients for clinical obesity in 2007 and a 2008 report from the NHS Information Centre claims that 'a third of children between the ages of 2 and 15 are now obese or overweight'. England has the fastest growing weight problem in Europe. The link between obesity and diabetes is well known and 100,000 UK patients are diagnosed with type 2 diabetes every year, fuelled by the nation's obesity problem. Douglas Smallwood, Chief Executive of the charity Diabetes UK says 'Diabetes is a serious condition which can lead to devastating complications such as blindness, amputation, heart and kidney disease.' Almost one hundred diabetics a week have a limb amputated because of complications with their disease.

An extra twelve kilograms in weight boosts the risk of cancer by 50%. Coronary heart disease causes 105,000 deaths a year and 2.6 million people are thought to be living with the symptoms of heart disease. Scientists have warned that unfit, lazy children are six times more likely to develop early signs of heart disease than those who are active and take exercise. For the first time, experts have established that activity levels in children as young as seven can have a serious effect on their future health. Professor Paul Gately, of Leeds Metropolitan University says 'Inactive children at a relatively young age are already storing up health risks for the future.' Health specialists, concerned for the health of our nation, are now repeatedly emphasising the importance of regular exercise as the best way to reduce the risks of suffering life-threatening illnesses in later life.

The National Obesity Forum has called for urgent action to tackle the obesity problem which, they calculate, causes 30,000 deaths each year and emphasises that the time to act is in childhood before irreversible damage has been done, and while lifelong habits can be learned. British Heart Foundation research found that taking 30 minutes of moderate exercise most days reduces the risk of an early death by more than a quarter. Diabetes UK warns that obesity is making a diabetes epidemic inevitable. Physical activity and a sensible diet are the best ways to reduce the risk of developing diabetes. The World Cancer Research Fund 2007 Report, produced by scientists and medical experts from around the world, tells us that most cancers are preventable by choosing a healthy diet, being physically active and maintaining a healthy weight. They recommend being physically active for at least 30 minutes every day, to keep the heart healthy and to reduce the risk of cancer.

Realistically, it is only in schools in physical education lessons, that we can encourage and help children to succeed in a wide range of physical skills and inspire, motivate and facilitate a joy in physical activity that will combat the health problems mentioned above. Physical education makes a unique contribution to an all-round, balanced education, but it also makes a special contribution to a life-prolonging, healthy lifestyle. For today's primary school children regular, excellent, vigorous and enjoyable physical education lessons are probably the best health products they will ever receive.

Teaching Physical Education

The teacher of physical education, almost uniquely, works alone and unaided, and is involved in whole class teaching with no help from the mass of teaching aids that help to keep pupils purposefully and often independently engaged in their classrooms. Even if he or she is talking to an individual, a pair or a small group, the teacher in a physical education lesson still needs to be aware of the whole class and how it is responding to the set task.

The teacher is the source and inspiration for everything that happens in the lessons. He or she needs to be well prepared to make the lesson complete, enjoyable, stimulating and challenging; enthusiastic to create an equally enthusiastic response; warm and encouraging to help pupils feel pleased and good about themselves; and intensely interested in inspiring vigorous physical activity in pupils, many of whom, away from school, may have inactive and sedentary lifestyles.

The lesson plan is the teacher's essential guide and reminder of the current lesson's content. Failure to plan and record lessons results in the same or similar things being done, month after month. Parts of the lesson gradually disappear, and an unprepared teacher can finish up doing no teaching in a lesson where everything is vague or has been done before. Pupils at apparatus in such an unprepared lesson answer 'Nothing' when asked 'What has your group been asked to do at this apparatus?'

July's lesson will only be at a more advanced stage that the previous September's if all the lessons in between have been recorded and referred to, to make each succeeding lesson move on and introduce new, interesting and exciting challenges. The lesson usually runs for four or five weeks (one lesson per week) to give the class enough time to practise, improve, develop, learn, remember and enjoy all the skills involved.

'Dead spots' and queue avoidance. The 'scenes of busy activity' which every physical education lesson should be requires an understanding by all pupils that they should be 'found working, not waiting'. This means that they need to be trained to respond immediately, behave well, keep on practising until stopped, and avoid standing immobile in queues.

The teacher needs to avoid talking the class out of their lesson through over-long explanations, demonstrations and pupil reflections following demonstrations. Lessons that lose a lot of time result in unsatisfactory, hurried apparatus work, frustratingly short time for playing games, and half-created dances with no time to share them proudly, with the class.

Demonstrations and observations by pupils and teacher are essential teaching aids because we remember what we see – good quality work; safe, correct ways to perform; the exact meanings of physical education terminology; and good examples of variety and interesting contrasts. All can watch one, two or a small group. Half of the class can watch the other half. Each can watch a partner. These occasional demonstrations, with comments by the observing pupils, often bring out good points not noticed by the teacher; train pupils to understand the elements of 'movement'; and let teachers ask 'how can it be improved?' Making friendly, encouraging, helpful points to classmates is good for class morale and for extending the class repertoire in physical education. ('Occasional' means once or twice at most in one lesson because of the time taken to do this.)

Further class practice should always follow a demonstration so that everyone can try to include some of the good features praised and commented on.

Shared choice or **indirect teaching** takes place when the teacher decides the nature of the activity and challenges the class to decide on the actions. Limits set are determined by the experience of the pupils. From the simple 'Can you travel on the apparatus, using your hands and feet?' with its slight limitations, we can progress on to 'Can you travel on the apparatus, using hands and feet, and include a still balance, a direction change, and taking all the weight on your hands at some point?'

Shared choice teaching produces a wide variety of results to add to the class repertoire. Being creative is extremely satisfying and most primary school pupils enjoy and are capable of making individual responses.

Direct teaching takes place when the teacher tells the class what to do, including, for example: any of the traditional gymnastic skills; the way to hold, throw and catch a ball; or how to do a folk dance step. Correct, safe ways to move; support yourself; grip, lift and carry apparatus; and throw implements, are all directly taught.

If the class is restless, not responding, or doing poor work, a directed activity can restore interest and discipline and provide ideas and a valuable starting point from which to develop. Pupils who are less interested, less inventive or less gifted physically, will benefit from direct teaching, particularly if the teacher can suggest an alternative, simpler but equally acceptable idea. 'If you do not like rolling forwards, try rolling sideways instead. Start, curled up on your back, with your hands clasped under your knees. This keeps your head out of the way.' The occasional stimulus of a direct request is the kind of challenge many pupils enjoy, and they respond enthusiastically. 'Can you and your partner bat the small ball up and down between you, six times?'

Motivational teaching. Children say that the things that motivate them to take part in physical activities are fun and skill development. They want to enjoy, learn and succeed. The more philosophical among them might also add that feelings of happiness are associated with having something to look forward to; to enjoy; and then to remember with pleasure (and often with pride). This anticipation, realisation and retrospect-inspiring potential of excellent physical education lessons and activities, makes it the favourite subject for many primary school pupils.

Safe Practice and Accident Prevention

In physical education lessons, where a main aim is to contribute to normal, healthy growth and physical development, we must do everything possible to avoid accidents.

Good supervision by the teacher is key to safe practice. He or she must be there with the class at all times, and teaching from positions from which the majority of the class can be seen. This usually means circulating on the outside looking in, with no-one behind his or her back. Good teaching develops skilful, well-controlled, safe movement with pupils wanting to avoid others to ensure that they have space to practise and perform well and not be impeded in any way. The outward expression of this caring attitude we are trying to create is the sensible, unselfish sharing of hall floor space, apparatus and playground, and self-control in avoiding others.

Badly behaved classes who do not respond immediately, or start or stop as requested; who rush around selfishly and noisily disturbing others; who are never quiet in their tongues or body movements; and who do not try to move well, are destructive of any prospects for high standards or lesson enjoyment by the majority and the teacher. A safe environment requires a well-behaved, quiet, attentive and responsive class. Good behaviour must be continually pursued until it becomes the normal, expected way to work in every lesson. There is nothing to talk about, apart from those occasions when comments are requested after a demonstration, or when partners are quietly discussing their response to a challenge.

The hall should be at a good working temperature with windows and doors opened or closed to cope with changing seasons and central heating variations. Potentially dangerous chairs, tables, trolleys, piano or television should be removed or pushed against a wall or into a corner. Floor sockets for receiving securing pins for ropes and climbing frames should be regularly cleared of cleaning substances which harden and block the small sockets.

In playground games lessons, pupils must be trained to remain inside the lines of the grids or netball courts and to avoid running, chasing or dodging into fences, walls, sheds, seats, hutted classrooms, or steps into buildings. In any 'tag' games, pupils must be told 'Touch the person you have caught very gently, never pushing them or causing them to fall or stumble.'

Before the lesson, the teacher checks for sensible, safe clothing with no watches, rings or jewellery whose impact against another child can cause serious scarring or injury; no long trousers that catch heels; no long sleeves that catch thumbs, impeding safe gripping; and no long, un-bunched hair that impedes vision. Indoors, barefoot work is recommended because it is quiet, provides a safe, strong grip on apparatus, enhances the appearance of the work, and enables the little-used muscles of feet and ankles to develop as they grip, balance, support, propel and receive the body weight.

In teaching gymnastic activities, the following safety considerations are important:

○ In floor and apparatus work, pupils need to be taught the correct, safe, 'squashy' landing after a jump so that they land safely on the balls of the feet, with ankles, knees and hips 'giving' without jarring.

○ When inverted, with all the weight on their hands, pupils need to be taught to keep fingers pointing forward, arms straight and strong, and head looking forward, not back under arms. Looking back under the arms makes every-thing appear to be upside down.

○ On climbing frames, pupils must be told 'Fingers grip over the bar, thumbs grip under the bar, always, for a safe, strong grip.'

Headings When Considering Standards in Physical Education

Physical Education lessons are so visual that most of the following headings can be considered by an interested observer.

○ **Vigorous physical activity**, involving all pupils for most of the lesson, is the most important feature of an excellent lesson.

○ **Responsive pupils, behaving well and obviously enjoying lessons**; working hard to learn and improve skills; and exuding enthusiasm and concentration, are an uplifting feature of high standards.

○ **Enthusiastic teaching, using praise and encouragement warmly**, stimulates pupils to even greater levels of endeavour. Praise is specific, referring to what is pleasing, to inform the pupil being praised and to let others hear and learn. 'Well done, Susan. Your balances are still, firm and beautifully stretched.'

○ **Skills, appropriate to the age group, are taught and developed**. There is an impression of skilful, quiet, confident, well-controlled, successful performing with economy of effort. Pupils show understanding by their ability to remember and repeat their movements.

○ **Pupils' behaviour towards one another is excellent**. Undressing and dressing quickly to extend lesson time; safe, unselfish sharing of space and apparatus; working quietly to avoid lessons being stopped because of noise; observing demonstrations with interest and then making helpful, friendly comments; and co-operating well as partners and members of groups and teams, all indicate desirable standards of behaviour.

○ **Varied teaching styles include**:

a indirect or shared choice teaching

b direct teaching

c good and varied use of demonstrations, observations, comments.

○ **Satisfactory time allocation** provides regular, weekly lessons in dance, games and gymnastic activities – a broad programme which also includes athletic activities and swimming for Juniors.

○ **Lesson plans** are in evidence, as a reminder of all parts of the current lesson, and as a reminder of what has been taught, so that the work can be progressed, month by month, throughout the year.

○ **Sensibly dressed pupils** wear shorts, a T shirt or blouse, and plimsolls. Indoors, barefoot work is recommended. As an example, the teacher should at least change into appropriate footwear.

○ **Continuity and progression from year to year** are evident in the way that older pupils work harder for longer at increasingly difficult activities, demonstrating skill and versatility.

○ **An awareness of safe practice and accident prevention** is evident in the way that pupils share the limited space. The correct way to lift, carry and use apparatus, land, move, roll, support and use the body generally, are regularly mentioned.

A Suggested Way to Start a First Lesson With a New Class

Unless taught otherwise, pupils travel round the hall or the playground in an anti-clockwise circle, all following the person in front of them. If one pupil slows down or stops suddenly, the next can bump into that person, possible knocking him or her over, causing an angry upset and a disturbance.

By travelling and confining themselves within this circle, a class fails to use all the possible room or playground space, depriving themselves of enough space to travel freely in different directions, and to join several actions together, on the spot or travelling about. Also, with everyone travelling round in a circle, sometimes side by side, pairs of less well-behaved pupils can be so close together that their poor behaviour, expressed in talking, not listening, slow responses, and noisy, poor performances, completely upsets the teacher's aim to give the class an enjoyable, lively, quiet, thoughtful and co-operative start to the lesson and the year's programme.

By continually making the whole class listen for the signal 'Stop!', we force them to pay attention, listen, and respond quickly.

Suggested pre-start to the lesson

1 Please show me your very best walking...go! Visit every part of the room, the sides, the ends, corners, as well as the middle. Swing your arms strongly and step out smartly.

2 When I call 'Stop!', show me how quickly you can stop and stand perfectly still. Keep walking smartly and visiting all parts of the room. Stop! Stand still!

3 If you are standing too near a piece of apparatus, like Liam by the piano, or too near someone else, like Thomas and Emily, please take one step into a big space all by yourself. Go!

4 When you start walking this time, travel along straight lines, never following anyone. If you find yourself behind someone, change direction and continue along a new straight line, following no-one. Ready? Go!

5 Come on. March briskly and smartly and pretend you are leaving footprints in every part of the room. When I call 'Stop!' you will stop immediately and then take a step into your own space if you are near apparatus or another person. Stop!

6 In our next practice, listen for my 'Stop!' and show me that no-one is standing behind another person, looking towards that person's back, following them. Go!

7 Stop! Stand still, after moving onto your own space if necessary. Now show your very best running, with the emphasis on lifting your heels, knees and hands to keep your running soft, silent and strong – and, of course, travelling along straight lines, never following anyone.

8 Stop! Be still! This half of the class stand with feet apart, arms folded, to watch this other half doing their very best running. Look out for and tell me later about anyone whose running you liked and be able to tell me what you liked about it. The running half...ready...go! Do not pick anyone who is following someone, or anyone who is not lifting heels, knees or arms strongly. Please watch carefully.

9 Stop! Watchers, whose running did you like. Yes, Daniel?

10 I (Daniel) liked Kate's running because she used her eyes well, looking for spaces, and she seemed to float along beautifully and easily, with heels, knees and hands being lifted high.

11 Thank you very much, Daniel, for that excellent answer. Now let's look at Kate to see and learn from the good things mentioned by Daniel. Please run again, Kate.

12 (Repeat with the other half working and the other half observing and commenting.)

Potential Cross-Curricular Outcomes of Physical Education Lessons for Juniors

Language Many teachers recognise the valuable contribution that physical education lessons can make to language development and a clearer understanding of the meanings of words. Hearing, reading and writing are the usual relationships between pupils and words. In physical education lessons, pupils do, experience and feel the action words concerned. Clear demonstrations by the teacher or a pupil also lead to a greater understanding of the exact meanings of action words.

In Year 3, Games Lesson 2, for example, there are: run, side-step, avoid, count, touch, walk, throw, catch, bounce, receive, pass, move, invent, develop, advance, change, practise, revise, show and skip. Jog, sprint, bowl, dodge, mark, chase, aim, reach, land, dribble and receive are also frequently used in games lessons.

In a typical gymnastic activities lesson, pupils will also experience, understand and feel the meanings of the many prepositions used, for example, in Year 4, Lesson 3: over, through, on, astride, along, upward, off, across, up to, from, near, away. Beside, beneath, towards, around, are also used frequently in gymnastics lessons.

Adverbs describe the quality or degree of effort in an action as in Year 5, Dance Lesson 9: vigorously, firmly, slowly, lively, lightly, loosely, stiffly, clearly and loudly. Quickly, gently, strongly, smoothly, suddenly, silently, smartly, carefully, splendidly and explosively, are also used frequently in dance lessons.

Writing Still within language, pupils can be challenged to complete 'The part(s) of the gymnastics lesson where I felt (choose one of) for example, excited, pleased, surprised, tired, proud, anxious, hot, breathless, strong, stretched, sociable, unsure, relaxed, was/were...' They can be asked to try to explain why they were experiencing the feelings that they listed.

A mountaineer once said 'When I climb, I can feel life effervescing within me.' A pupil who has just completed a rope climb for the first time; or done a beautifully controlled handstand, then lowered into a forward roll; or completed their own created dance or gymnastic sequence with complete control from start to finish, with attractive use of space and effort; or outwitted a close marking opponent, before going on to score, will be experiencing intense excitement, pride and pleasure, deserving of the opportunity to try to produce an eloquent expression about what might have been an unforgettable event.

Art They can be asked 'Can you draw the gymnastic action or actions that gave you the most pleasure or excitement in today's lesson? Under your heading, can you explain in a few words why you were pleased or excited?'

Physical Education can also contribute to pupils':

○ **spiritual development** through helping them gain a sense of achievement and develop positive attitudes towards themselves

○ **moral development** through helping pupils gain a sense of fair play based on rules and the conventions of activities; and develop positive sporting behaviour, knowing how to conduct themselves in sporting competition

○ **social development** through helping pupils develop social skills in activities involving co-operation and collaboration, responsibility, personal commitment, loyalty and teamwork, and considering the social importance of physical activity, sport and dance.

Gymnastic Activities

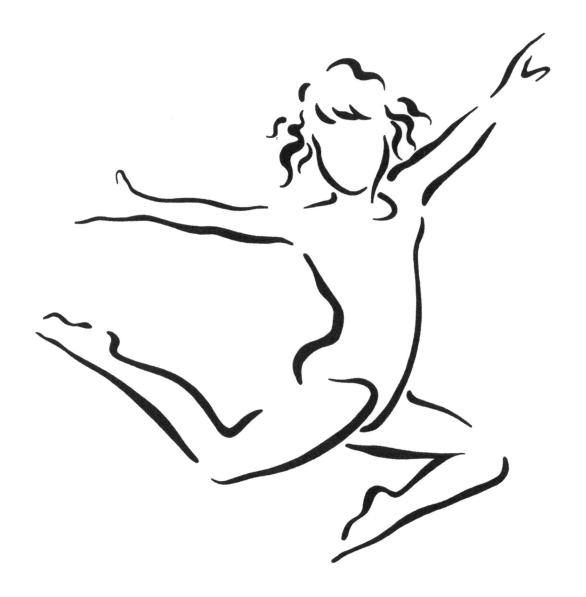

Introduction to Gymnastic Activities

Gymnastic Activities is the indoor lesson that includes varied floorwork on a clear floor, unimpeded by apparatus, followed by varied apparatus work which should take up just over half of the lesson time. Ideally, the portable apparatus will have been positioned around the sides and ends of the room, near to where it will be used, before lessons start in the morning or afternoon. This allows each of the seven or eight mixed infant groups, or the five or six mixed junior groups of pupils to lift, carry and position their apparatus in a very short time, because no set will need to be moved more than 3-5 metres. The lesson is traditionally of 30 minutes duration.

The following pages aim, first of all, to produce a sense of staff-room unity regarding the nature of good practice and high standards in teaching Gymnastic Activities lessons. Without this sense of unity among the teachers concerned, there is no continuity of aims, expectations or programme, and there will be a less than satisfactory level of achievement. Secondly, the following pages provide a full scheme of work for Gymnastic Activities. There is a lesson plan and accompanying pages of detailed explanatory notes for every month, designed to help teachers and schools with ideas for lessons that are progressive.

Why We Teach Gymnastic Activities

Ideally, the expressions of intent known as 'Aims' should represent the combined views of all the staff.

Aim 1 To inspire vigorous physical activity to promote normal healthy growth and physical development. Physical Education is most valuable when pupils' participation is enthusiastic, vigorous and wholehearted. All subsequent aims for a good programme depend on achieving this first aim.

Aim 2 To teach physical skills to develop skilful, well-controlled, versatile movement. We want pupils to enjoy moving well, safely and confidently. Physical Education makes a unique contribution to a child's physical development because the activities are experienced at first hand by doing them.

Aim 3 To help pupils become good learners as well as good movers. Knowledge, understanding and learning are achieved through a combination of doing, feeling and experiencing physical activity. Pupils are challenged to think for themselves, making decisions about their actions.

Aim 4 To develop pupils' self-confidence and self-esteem by appreciating the importance of physical achievement; by helping them to achieve; and by recognising and sharing such achievement with others.

Aim 5 To develop desirable social qualities, helping pupils get on well with one another by bringing them together in mutual endeavours. Friendly, co-operative, close relationships are an ever-present feature of Physical Education lessons.

Aim 6 To provide opportunities for exciting, almost adventurous actions (particularly climbing, swinging, balancing, jumping and landing) and vigorous exercise – seldom experienced away from school. We want our pupils to use these lessons as outlets for their energy and we want them to believe that exercise is good for you and your heart, and makes you feel and look better. We aim to encourage participation in a healthy lifestyle, long after pupils have left school.

The Gymnastic Activities Lesson Plan for Juniors – 30–35 minutes

One answer to the question 'What do we teach in a gymnastic activities lesson?' might be – 'All the natural actions and ways of moving of which the body is capable and which, if practised wholeheartedly and safely, ensure normal, healthy growth and physical development.'

It has been said that 'What you don't use, you lose.' Most pupils hardly ever use their natural capacity for vigorous running; jumping and landing from a height; rolling in a different direction; balancing on a variety of body parts; upending to take their weight on their hands; gripping, climbing and swinging on a rope; hanging, swinging or circling on a bar; or whole body bending, stretching, arching and twisting.

These natural movements and actions should be present in every gymnastic activities lesson, ensuring that pupils do not lose the ability to do them and have their physical development diminished.

A teacher's determination to inspire the class to use and not lose their natural physicality can be strengthened by observing how many children are collected in cars at the school gates. They are then transported home to their after school, house-bound, sedentary home lives.

Floorwork (12–15 minutes) starts the lesson and includes:

○ Activities for the legs, exploring and developing the many actions possible when travelling on feet, and ways to jump and land.

○ Activities for the body, including the many ways to bend, stretch, rock, roll, arch, twist, curl, turn, and the ways in which body parts receive, support and transfer the body weight in travelling and balancing.

○ Activities for the arms and shoulders, the least used parts of our body. We strengthen them by using them to hold all or part of the body weight on the spot or moving. This strength is needed in gripping, climbing, hanging, swinging and circling, and in levering on to and across apparatus, supported by the hands alone.

Apparatus Work (16–18 minutes) is the climax of the lesson, making varied, unique and challenging physical demands on pupils whose whole body – legs, arms and shoulders, back and abdominal muscles – has to work hard because of the more difficult tasks:

○ travelling on hands and feet, over, under, across and around obstacles, as well as vertically, often supported only on hands

○ jumping and landing from greater heights

○ rolling on to, along, from and across apparatus

○ balancing on high or narrow surfaces

○ upending to take all body weight on hands on apparatus above floor level

○ gripping, swinging, climbing and circling on ropes and bars.

Final Floor Activity (2 minutes) after the apparatus has been returned to its starting places around the sides, ends and corners of the hall, brings the whole class together again in a simple activity based on the lesson's main emphasis or theme. After the bustle of apparatus removal – the swishing of ropes along trackways, the creaking of climbing frames being wheeled away, the bumping of benches, planks, boxes and trestles – there is a quiet, calm, thoughtful and focused ending.

Three Ways to Teach Apparatus Work

1 **(Easiest Method) Pupils use all the apparatus freely, as they respond to tasks that relate to the lesson theme**. Several challenges provide non-stop apparatus work for infants and juniors. Pupils are stationary only when watching a demonstration, having a teaching point emphasised, or when being given the next task. This method is normally used with infant classes, because they are able to visit and use all pieces of apparatus, including their favourites – ropes and climbing frames.

   'Show me a still balance and beautifully stretched body shape on each piece of apparatus.' (Body shape awareness and balance)

   'Show me how you can approach each piece of apparatus going forward and leave going sideways.' (Space awareness – directions)

   'Leader, show your partner one touch only on each piece of apparatus, then off to the next piece.' (Partner work)

2 **Groups stay and work at one set of apparatus**. Repetition helps pupils improve and remember a series of linked actions. The task is the same for all groups, based on the lesson theme.

   'Make your hands important in arriving on, and your feet important in leaving the apparatus.' (Body parts awareness)

   'Can you include swings on to and off apparatus; a swing into a roll; and a swing to take all the weight on your hands?' (Swinging)

   'Travel from opposite sides, up to, on, along and from the apparatus, to finish in your partner's starting place.' (Partner work)

   Groups rotate to the next apparatus after about five minutes and will work at three sets in a lesson, rotating clockwise one lesson, and anti-clockwise the next, to meet all apparatus every two lessons.

3 **Each group practises a different, specific skill on each piece of apparatus - balancing, rolling, climbing, for example**. This method of teaching is more difficult than the other two because it needs more technical knowledge, and because the teacher is giving five or six sets of instructions instead of one. As it is a direct challenge to 'skills hungry' pupils, it is very popular.

   Benches 'At upturned benches, slowly balance and walk forward. Look straight ahead. Feel for the bench before you step on it.'

   Ropes 'Grip strongly with hands together and feet crossed. Can you take one hand off, while swinging, to prove a good foot grip?'

   Low cross box 'A face vault is like a high bunny jump to cross the box, as you twist over, facing the box top all the way.'

   Climbing frames 'Travel by moving hands only, then feet only.'

   Mats 'Roll sideways with body curled small and then with body long and stretched' (log roll).

   Groups rotate to the next piece of apparatus after about five minutes, rotating clockwise one lesson, and anti-clockwise the next lesson, meeting all apparatus every two lessons.

Organising Groups For Junior School Apparatus Work

Groups of five or six pupils are appropriate for junior school apparatus work, and pupils are placed in their mixed groups in the first lesson in September. Pupils are told 'These are your groups and starting places for apparatus work.' For the four or five sessions' development of a lesson, the same groups go to the same starting places, becoming more expert in lifting, carrying and placing their apparatus in that position.

From their regular starting positions, groups rotate clockwise, probably with time to work at three different sets of apparatus. At the end of the apparatus work, groups return to their own apparatus to move it back to the sides and ends of the room from which it was originally carried. The floor is now clear for the incoming class. In the next lesson, the groups will move anti-clockwise to work at the other three sets of apparatus.

This recommended system for ensuring that apparatus can be lifted, carried and placed in position quickly and easily, needs the co-operation of all the teachers. Before the lessons start in the morning or afternoon, the portable apparatus is placed around the sides and ends of the hall adjacent to where it will be used. Each group will only have to carry it 2–3 metres. A well-trained class can have the apparatus in place in 30 seconds. After all lessons are finished each day, as much of the apparatus as possible should remain in the hall, in corners, against or on the platform, or at the sides and ends of the room. Mats can be stored vertically behind frames, benches and boxes.

Positioning of Apparatus During Lessons

The teacher needs to provide varied actions and different physical demands as pupils progress from apparatus to apparatus to meet a challenging, interesting series of tasks which include:

a climbing and swinging on ropes

b rolling on mats, from benches, along low box

c balancing on inverted benches, planks, along low box

d running and jumping on to mats, across, along and from benches

e climbing on climbing frames

f taking weight on hands on mats, benches, planks, low boxes

g jumping and landing from a height from a bench or box

h circling or hanging from metal pole between trestles

i lying and pulling along a bench or down an inclined plank.

A safe environment is ensured by providing:

a mats where pupils are expected to land from a height

b mats that are well away from walls, windows, doors or other obstacles such as a piano, trolleys or chairs, and well away from the landing areas of adjacent apparatus

c height and width of apparatus that are appropriate for the age of the class – not too narrow to balance on, and not too high to jump from.

Mats are used to cushion a landing from a height and to roll on. We do not need mats under ropes or around climbing frames because we do not ask pupils to jump down from a height. If mats are placed around climbing frames, pupils often behave in a foolhardy way, enticed into dangerous jumping.

Fixed and portable apparatus

In the lesson plans that follow, the equipment continually being referred to and shown in the apparatus layouts includes the following items:

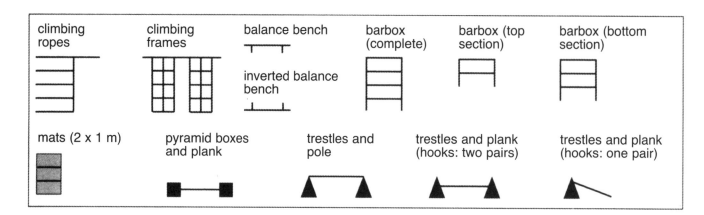

Minimum number recommended:

○ 12 × mats (2 × 1 m]

○ 3 × balance benches

○ 1 × barbox that can be divided into two smaller boxes by lifting off the top section; the remaining lower section should have a platform fitted

○ 1 × pair pyramid boxes and one plank

○ 1 × pair of 0.9 m, 1 m, and 1.4 m trestles

○ 1 metal pole to join pairs of trestles

○ 2 planks with two pairs of hooks

○ 2 planks with one pair of hooks

A Pattern for Teaching and Improving a Gymnastic Activities Action

Using 'Travelling' as an example

1 **Quickly into action**. With few words, clearly explain the task and challenge the class to start. For example 'Can you plan to travel, using your feet, sometimes going forwards, and sometimes in another direction?'

2 **While class is working**. Emphasise the main points, one at a time. There is no need to stop a well-behaved class who are working quietly every time you need to make a teaching point. 'Find quiet spaces in all parts of the room – the sides, ends, corners, as well as the middle.' 'Work so quietly that I can't hear you.' 'Travel on straight lines, never curving round, following someone.' 'Look over your shoulder if going backwards.'

3 **Identify and praise good work while class is working**. The teacher needs to circulate round the outside of the room, looking in to see as much of the work as possible. 'Well done, Thomas. I liked your skipping forwards and bouncing sideways.' 'Maisie, your hopscotch is a great idea.' 'Sarah, your slow, careful running backwards with high knees lifting, is a neat, safe way to travel.'

4 **Demonstrations accompanied by teacher comment are the quickest way to increase the class repertoire**. It saves time if the demonstrators have been told what aspect of movement they are about to be asked to demonstrate. 'We will be looking at your beautifully stretched body in your jumps, and the soft, quiet way you let your knees and ankles give when you land.' 'Stop and watch Daniel's lively, quiet bouncing with feet parting and closing, going sideways. And look at Charlotte's galloping backwards with a strong arm swing.'

   Beware of stopping the class too often to use a demonstration. Make these stoppages brief, between 12 and 15 seconds.

5 **Further practice should follow a demonstration with reminders of the good things seen**. Pupils enjoy copying something they never thought of trying – particularly when it has been warmly praised and approved of. 'Thank you for those excellent demonstrations. Practise again, and try to improve your travelling by using something of what you have just seen. Use your whole body strongly, but quietly. Your feet can travel together or apart, or one after the other.'

6 **Demonstrations (by an individual, a small group or half of the class) with follow-up comments by the pupils are used to let pupils reflect on and evaluate their own and others' performances**. Such comments and judgements guide the next stage of planning for improvement. 'Watch this group of four working and tell me which travelling actions you like best, and say which directions you saw being used.' This is followed by a brief look at the pupils mentioned.

7 **Demonstrators and those making comments are thanked and more class practice lets them try some of the good things seen**. Beware of using demonstrations with follow-up comments more than once or twice in the lesson because they are time-consuming.

Progressing Gymnastic Activities over the 4 or 5 weeks of the Lesson's Development

Using 'Stepping' as an example of an activity to be developed

Lessons 1 and 2

a Concentrate on the '**What?**', the actions, their correct form, and how the body parts concerned are working.

'Can you step quietly and neatly, visiting all parts of the room? Travel on straight lines, never following anyone.'

'Which parts of the foot can support you? Tip toes, insides or outsides? Long or short steps or a mixture?'

'Can you vary the idea of stepping, not always passing your feet?' (Chasse, crossover, toes down and swing.)

b Insist on good, clear body shapes to make everything look better and be more demanding.

'Step out nice and tall as you travel. Can you show me your clear arms, legs and body shape? Are you long and stretched or is there a body shape change somewhere?'

Lessons 2 and 3

Concentrate on the '**Where?**' of the movement, adding variety and quality by good use of own and whole floor space, directions and levels.

'Can you sometimes step on the spot, (particularly when you are in a crowded area) and sometimes use the whole room space – sides, corners, ends as well as middle.'

'Stepping actions sideways and backwards can be interesting – sliding, stepping-closing (chasse) or cross-stepping over, as well as feet passing normally. The leading leg can swing in many directions.'

Lessons 3 and 4

Consider the '**How?**' of the movements and the way that changes of speed and effort (force) might make the work look more controlled and neat, as well as giving them greater variety, contrast and interest.

'Within your stepping, can you include a change of speed? It might be slow, slow; quick, quick, 3, 4; slow, slow. Flat, flat; tip toes, tip toes, 3, 4; flat, flat.. This is interesting if a change of direction accompanies the speed change. Side, slow, slow; forward, quick, quick, 3, 4; side, slow, slow.' 'Can you make parts of your travelling small, soft, quiet, and make parts bigger, firmer, stronger?' (On the spot, keep it soft, 1, 2, 3, 4; on the move, big strong strides, 1, 2, 3, 4.)

Lessons 4 or Lessons 4 and 5

Ask for **sequences** that draw together all the practising, learning, adapting and remembering that have taken place during the previous lessons and aim for almost non-stop action, working harder for longer with enthusiasm, understanding and concentration.

'In your 3 or 4 part sequence, can you include: varied stepping actions, interesting use of space, and a change of speed or force somewhere?'

The Use of Themes in Teaching Gymnastic Activities

Week after week, month after month, the teacher and class come into the school hall and see the same apparatus, apparently offering the same limited set of activities every time. In dance, we continually move on to learning and performing new dances and building a huge repertoire. In games, the new seasons bring their different sports and the varied games implements provide an interesting and exciting range – including new games created by the teacher and pupils.

Gymnastic activities lessons are made different through applying a new idea, emphasis or theme each month. We do not simply 'do' the basic action. We do it, focusing on a particular aspect of movement, to improve in understanding and versatility, as well as in competence. A theme is a particular aspect of movement chosen by the teacher as a focal point around which to build a series of lessons.

At the very beginning of the series of four or five lessons during which an individual lesson is repeated, it is recommended that the pupils are 'put in the picture' regarding their lesson's main aims or emphases. In cases where they are going to be assessed on the outcome of the lesson, it is essential to explain to them what new skills, knowledge and understanding they will be expected to demonstrate. Identifying the lesson theme or main emphasis to the class is also a way for the teacher to put him or herself 'in the picture' about the main objectives of the lesson and to focus on them.

Start of year themes with a new class, will have an emphasis on good behaviour; sensible, safe sharing of floor and apparatus space; immediate responses to commands and challenges set by the teacher; establishing a tradition of wholehearted, vigorous effort and a co-operative attitude towards one's classmates; and co-operating with others to lift, carry and place apparatus quietly, sensibly and safely.

A suggested set of six progressive themes for a month to month programme

1   **Body parts awareness** for better controlled, safer, more correct activity. 'Show me varied ways to travel, using one foot, both feet, or one foot after the other.'

2   **Body shape awareness** for improved poise, better posture and firmer body tension. 'Can you run and jump up high with feet together and long, straight legs?'

3   **Space awareness** for improved variety, quality and interest, and safer practising. 'Can you travel all round the room, using feet only, sometimes going forwards, and sometimes sideways?'

4   **Effort awareness** for more interesting contrasts, better quality and stronger work. 'As you travel in a variety of ways can you include actions that are small, light and gentle, and actions that are large, lively and strong?'

5   **Sequences** for longer, harder, versatile work, stamping it with own personality. 'Make up a sequence you can remember, of three or four joined-up actions and changing body shapes on different body parts.' (Standing, kneeling, lying, sitting, upended on shoulders, arched on back or front.)

6   **Partner work** for new, enjoyable, sociable, more demanding experiences not possible on one's own, and to extend movement understanding because you need to recognise partner's actions. 'Stand, facing each other. Can you, with a little bend of knees as a start signal, bounce at the same speed? Can you do opposites, with one going up as the other comes down?'

A Progressive Series of Themes for a Gymnastic Activities Programme

An example from parts of lessons based on 'ways to travel'

Floorwork

Apparatus Work

Theme 1. Body parts awareness – for neater, better controlled, safer, more correct activity.

a Show me varied ways to travel, using one foot, both feet, or one foot after the other. As you travel about, slowly, using hands and feet, can you make different parts of your body go first?

a Plan to visit many pieces of apparatus. 'Feel' the different ways your hands and feet can:
  1 support you (for example, as you hang, swing, crawl, circle, roll, slide, skip, jump, balance.)
  2 go from apparatus to apparatus, putting hands on the apparatus, and show me a bunny jump with straight arms and well bent legs.

Theme 2. Body shape awareness – for improved poise, better posture and firmer body tension.

a Can you run and jump up high with feet together and long, straight legs?

b Can you run and jump up high to show me a wide shape like a star?

a Run quietly round the room, not touching any apparatus. When I call 'Stop!', show me a clear body shape on the nearest apparatus.

b Run round again and when I stop you next time, show me a different, firm body shape.

Theme 3. Space awareness – for improved variety, quality and interest, and safer practising.

a Can you travel all round the room, using feet only, sometimes forwards, and sometimes going sideways? Which are best for going forwards? Which are best for going sideways?

a Can you arrive on and leave the apparatus at different places and in different ways?

b Take weight on hands, with straight arms and bent legs. Bring feet down slowly in a new floor space.

Theme 4. Effort awareness – for more interesting contrasts, better quality, and stronger work.

As you travel in a variety of ways, can you include actions that are small, light and gentle, and actions that are large, lively and strong?

Travel freely. Show me strong, firm balances on apparatus that contrast with easier travelling actions in between. Can you do a vigorous upward jump, off, then a soft 'giving' landing.

Theme 5. Sequences – for longer, harder, versatile work, stamping it with own personality.

Work in a small floor space and show me two or more ways to travel on feet or feet and hands. Can you give each action a name? Show me a still start and finish.

Start in a still, nicely balanced position on the floor. Travel on to a piece of apparatus and show me a neat, still balance position.

Theme 6. Partner work – for new, more exciting experiences not possible on your own.

Follow your leader's varied travelling.

Follow on to and along each piece of apparatus.

National Curriculum Requirements for Gymnastic Activities – Key Stage 2: The Main Features

'The government believes that two hours of physical activity a week, including the National Curriculum for Physical Education and extra-curricular activities, should be an aspiration for all schools. This applies to all stages.'

Programme of study *Pupils should be taught to:*

a   create and perform fluent sequences on the floor and using apparatus

b   include variations in level, speed and directions in their sequences.

Attainment target *Pupils should be able to demonstrate that they can:*

a   link skills, techniques and ideas and apply them appropriately, showing precision, control and fluency

b   compare and comment on skills, techniques and ideas used in own and others' work and use this understanding to improve their own performances by modifying and refining skills and techniques.

Main NC headings when considering assessment, achievement and progression

○ **Planning** – in a focused, thoughtful, safe way, thinking ahead to an intended outcome. Evidence of satisfactory planning can be seen in:

   a   good decision-making, sensible, safe judgements and good understanding of what was asked for

   b   an understanding of the elements that enhance quality, variety and contrast in 'movement'

   c   the expression of personal qualities such as optimism, enthusiasm, and a capacity for hard work in pursuit of improvement.

○ **Performing and improving performance** successfully is the main aim. In a satisfactory performance a pupil demonstrates:

   a   well-controlled, neat and accurate work, concentrating on the main feature of the task

   b   the ability to practise to improve skilfulness, performing safely

   c   whole-hearted and vigorous activity, sharing the space sensibly and unselfishly, with a concern for own and others' safety

   d   the ability to remember and repeat actions.

○ **Linking actions** – as pupils build longer, more complex sequences of linked actions in response to the stimuli, demonstrating that they are:

   a   working harder for longer, showing a clear beginning, middle and end to their sequence

   b   pursuing almost non-stop, vigorous and enjoyable action.

○ **Reflecting and evaluating** – as pupils describe what they and others have done, say what they liked about a performance, give an opinion on how it might be improved; and then make practical use of such reflection to plan again to improve.

Year 6 Gymnastic Activities Programme

Pupils should be able to:

Autumn	Spring	Summer
1 Re-establish good traditions of enjoyment, safety and achievement – quick responses to instructions; good sharing of floor and apparatus; working hard to improve.	**1** Adopt good posture always and use body safely and sensibly in lifting and carrying, jumping and landing, rolling and up-ending.	**1** Recognise the importance of, and value, an active lifestyle. 'What you don't use, you lose.'
2 Work vigorously to develop strength and suppleness, and to exercise heart and lungs.	**2** Respond imaginatively to challenges, doing one's best to produce quiet, neat, controlled work with enthusiasm.	**2** Understand the value of, and be able to sustain, vigorous physical activity.
3 Demonstrate originality and versatility in neat, controlled work.	**3** Understand the value of and demonstrate sustained activity.	**3** Revise and improve traditional skills; mat agilities; circles and climbs on a rope; balances on inverted benches; circling on bars; head and handstands.
4 Explore different means of rolling, balancing, jumping.	**4** Work and practise hard, with determination, until a task is mastered.	**4** Make appropriate decisions quickly in planning responses.
5 Improve skills of rope climbing; travelling on hands and feet; rolling; balancing.	**5** Emphasise changes of shape with a constant concern for good-looking, poised movements.	**5** Plan longer sequences, able to envisage the finished product, and showing aesthetic qualities, including contrast, variety and repetition.
6 Enhance sequences by including contrasts of shape, speed, effort, direction or level.	**6** Be space aware, expressed in changes of direction and level, and varied use of own and the general shared space.	**6** Observe, copy, contrast or match a partner's movements, developing one's powers of observation and an awareness of the elements of movement.
7 Plan and perform, knowing, for example, start and finish places; places to jump, to roll and to balance.	**7** Demonstrate good use of effort to achieve a well-controlled performance.	**7** Plan appropriate solutions, sometimes imaginatively, to the various challenges encountered.
8 Improve body-parts awareness, understanding how hands, feet and larger parts carry, support, propel, grip and act generally.	**8** Display understanding, generally, by its effect on planning.	**8** Improve, refine and repeat a series of movements performed previously, with increasing control and accuracy.
9 Plan, practise, improve and remember more complex sequences.	**9** Refine and adapt performance when working with a partner.	**9** Make judgements about own and others' performance, and use this information to improve the accuracy, quality and variety of performance.
10 Appraise a sequence of movement using relevant terminology.	**10** Perform with a sense of commitment.	
	11 Recognise when a sequence is appropriate to the aims of the performer.	

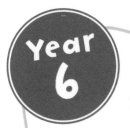
Lesson Plan 1 • 30-35 minutes
September

Theme: *Re-establishing those essential traditions without which the optimum levels of enjoyment, safety and achievement will never be realised: (a) all reacting immediately to the teacher's instructions; (b) all unselfishly sharing floor and apparatus space to promote safety and good working conditions; (c) all contributing to a co-operative, quiet, working atmosphere.*

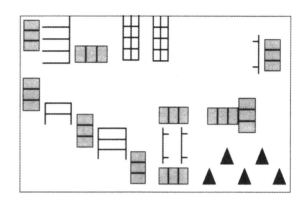

Floorwork
12—15 minutes

Legs

1   Can you change quietly and smoothly between running and other activities such as walking, running and skipping?

2   Can you change, also, between actions on the spot, when your floor is crowded, and movements when you travel more widely when space permits? Keep looking as you move.

Body

1   Can you travel, going from a wide body shape to a new wide shape?

2   You can be standing; lying; on hands and feet; with one side to floor on one hand and foot.

Arms

1   Which parts of your body can give you a swing up on to hands?

2   Try long arms starting above head; one foot kicking up behind you; one arm leading into a cartwheel; two arms and one leg.

Apparatus Work
16—18 minutes

1   Walk quietly all around the room, touching floor and mats, and keeping well away from all others.

2   Change to your best running, carefully weaving in and out of apparatus and others. When I call 'Stop!' show me a wide shape on the nearest piece of apparatus. Stop!

3   Stay at your number one apparatus to practise, improve and remember the following.

Climbing frames
Make short travels into a balance, particularly trying to show a 'firm', wide body shape.

Ropes, mats
Revise rope climbing, saying to yourself 'Hand, hand, hands together, feet up', aiming for a stretched body after the three hand movements.

Trestles
Find as many parts of the trestles, or trestles and floor, as possible, to balance on.

Benches, mats
a   Can you make your hands important in travelling along or across the benches?
b   Show me ways to go from benches on to mats.

Cross bench, mats
Drive up and off the cross bench using one or both feet. At return mats, can you show me a balance, roll, balance sequence?

Boxes, mats
Face vault, i.e. 'bunny jump', over the low, cross boxes.

Final Floor Activity
2 minutes

Travel on legs and swing up into a turn to a still landing, using arms well for balance.

Teaching notes and NC guidance
Development over 4 lessons

NC elements being emphasised:

a Exploring different means of taking weight on hands.
b Being physically active.
c Responding to instructions.

Floorwork

Legs

1 Running has to link pairs of other activities. One of the activities can be slow as you look for a space, for your run into the third activity which can be more lively.

2 Pupils seldom practise working on the spot, when there is a sudden crowding. Every leg activity can be performed in your own space which provides an attractive contrast to the free movement.

Body

1 From wide to wide shape is unusual and quite difficult. A directed start by the teacher will help to get everyone moving. From the directed start, week by week, they can add and develop their own ideas for supporting parts and linking movements.

2 The standing high level; medium level, arched on hands and feet; and the low level side falling with one side towards floor, on one hand and one foot, provide a good example of varied levels.

Arms

1 They will have gone up on to hands hundreds of times, possibly without thinking about where the impetus is coming from.

2 Long arms swing from above head is a slow, powerful, long lever action used by most pupils to start with. The one foot swing/kick up behind body gives a quick, neat, more easily controlled swing.

Apparatus Work

1 The floor circulation, without touching any apparatus, is an exercise in sharing the floor, keeping well away from others, not all following one another around or queuing.

2 'Stop!' is an exercise in 'reacting immediately to instructions', setting a standard of responsiveness for the year.

Climbing frames
Balances look better and are harder physically when we stretch out fully the parts not supporting us.

Ropes
Revise, if necessary, the strong, crossed feet grip position, with sole over instep, that grips you when you take one hand off to climb up.

Trestles
One foot and hand; two hands; two feet; lying on tummy, plus many balances using floor and part of trestle.

Benches, mats
Pull along on back or front; bunny jump or cartwheel across; feet off and on alternately as hands support along; jump feet between or astride to standing on, jump off.

Cross bench, mats
The vigorous run and spring off bench can contrast with the more restrained balance, roll, balance.

Boxes, mats
Hands on box; bunny jump up with high hips; twist around to land, facing box all the time in the face vault.

Final Floor Activity

A short 3–4 metres travel into a swing up into a turn can be done back and forwards in own, small corridor.

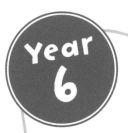

Year 6

Lesson Plan 2 • 30-35 minutes
October

Theme: *Re-establishing the tradition of quiet, varied, thoughtful, continuous work. Good spacing to prevent frustration and allow safe practice is also being strongly emphasised.*

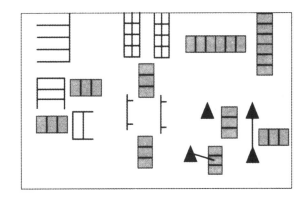

Floorwork
12—15 minutes

Legs

1   Can you run and jump high, run and jump long, using good arm and leg positions to help you balance in flight and on landing?

2   What take-off actions of feet help long and high jumps?

3   What arm positions best help you to balance on landing?

Body

1   Practise and link together any big body movements while standing, upended on shoulders, or with your front, back or side to the floor.

2   Body movements include curling, arching, stretching, twisting.

Arms

Still thinking of natural body movements, can you travel, slowly, with your weight on your hands, or hands and feet, by changing body shape?

Apparatus Work
16—18 minutes

Climbing frames
Climb vertically. Try to twist down, legs leading, using hands and arms only for support. Use crossed hands grip, sitting on top bar, one hand gripping towards you, the other gripping with knuckles away from you. Lower body by rotating to near hand side.

Ropes
Use two ropes to show a sequence that includes curling, circling and hanging upside down.

Upturned benches
Cat walk along upturned bench on all fours with weight evenly distributed between hands and feet, with knees and hips low. As a contrast, balance with body tall and stretched. While waiting your turn on the benches try some other balancing on the mats (e.g. elbow balance or bent leg headstand).

Boxes, mat
Can you cross the cross box using hands only? Can you return along the long box, using legs only?

Mats
Revise and expand your floorwork sequence of linked large body movements. Working on the mats means that you can be a bit more adventurous (e.g. rolls can be more comfortably used as ways to link movements together).

Final Floor Activity
2 minutes

Can you plan and show me a triangle of three jumps back to your starting position? Make one high, one long and one of your choice (e.g. tucked, jacknife, star).

Teaching notes and NC guidance
Development over 4 lessons

NC elements being emphasised:

a Exploring, developing, practising, refining and repeating a longer series of actions, making increasingly complex sequences on floor and using apparatus.

b Working vigorously to develop suppleness and strength, and to exercise the heart and lungs strongly.

Floorwork

Legs

1 Plan start and finish positions on floor. Plan to do runs and jumps, there and back to starting place, or to move around room.

2 Long jump is helped by one-footed takeoff. High jump is helped by two-footed takeoff. You can land with feet together or apart, or with one foot arriving after the other, slowing you down.

3 Stretched arms give good shape and help balance, usually stretched to front or to sides.

Body

1 Pretend you are in a large bubble and try to push its sides away from you, stretched or wide.

2 'Big' means involving whole of body which includes big outwards as in stretching, or a big curl, tightly inwards.

Arms

Ask for slow, careful whole body movements, not quick little scampering where body weight is mostly on feet anyway. Long crawls until body is almost horizontal; bunny jumps with shoulders over hips over hands; cat springs (flight from feet on to hands); bouncing with whole body coming up off floor; crab; cartwheels.

Apparatus Work

Climbing frames

Thumbs are curled under bars for a safe, strong grip. The 'rotary travelling' descent is a strong arms and abdominals action.

Ropes

When circling or hanging upside down, it is important to grip rope at shoulder height with bent arms to ensure feet return safely to standing on floor.

Upturned benches

In cat walk, centre of gravity must be kept low with knees well down below level of bench. Hand, hand, foot, foot travel with a strong hand grip. Feet are balanced on top of bench.

Boxes, mats

In crossing box with hands only, experiment by approaching box from front, at an angle, and even side towards. One or both hands can support you, and you can cross with back towards the box.

Mats

A moving 'bubble' of large body movements, now on mats, can include handstands, cartwheels, crab arches and dive rolls.

Final Floor Activity

The interesting variety provided by the different shapes can be expanded by varied take-offs and landing actions in the jumps. Take-off can be from one or both feet. Landings can be on to both feet together or apart, or on to one foot, then the other for a slower, controlled finish.

Year 6

Lesson Plan 3 • 30-35 minutes
November

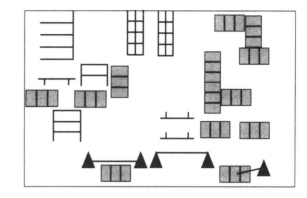

Theme: *Jumping and landing, rolling and balancing.*

Floorwork
12—15 minutes

Legs

1 Show me a beautifully stretched and balanced starting position on tiptoes or on one foot. Run a few steps and swing up into a high jump with a turn in flight or on landing. Finish, beautifully stretched and balanced.

2 How are you holding your arms to help balance in flight and on landing?

3 A landing with feet astride, or one foot landing after the other, slowly, also helps to control your finish.

Body

1 Log roll. With feet tight together, body fully stretched and arms stretched upwards, show me a sideways roll with your straight body.

2 Circle roll. Start, sitting in the straddle position, with feet wide apart. Move sideways, keeping legs wide apart and straight as you lower on to back. Keep your piked hips, hold your shape as you continue to roll sideways on your back. Finish, having made a half-turn, to face the opposite way.

Arms

1 Put both hands on the floor under your shoulders. Do three little preparatory bounces of feet off floor, keeping arms straight and head looking forwards. On the fourth big bounce go up into your bunny jump with knees kept well bent.

2 Remembering that bent leg position, try a handstand where you let bent legs 'dangle' down over head, helping balance.

Apparatus Work
16—18 minutes

1 Use all the floor and apparatus freely to show me:

a a still, ready position on tiptoes;

b a short run and jump into a turn on landing in balance;

c a roll on mats or floor;

d a balance on any piece or pieces of apparatus.

2 At your starting apparatus position, practise, improve and remember the following.

Climbing frames
Show me a balance: using floor and frame; with body through one of the spaces; and on one outside of the frame.

Ropes
Climb after a strong upward jump to place both hands high and together, or run and jump into a strong swing which ends in a well balanced landing.

Trestles
Can you show me parts of the apparatus where you can hold a 'firm' stretched balance on three body parts, then two body parts, then one body part?

Inverted benches, trestle
Bent leg head-stand on the mats. Hands and forehead placed on mat to make a triangle. With weight equally on forehead and hands, feet walk in to raise hips above point of support. Knees bend to raise feet from floor.

Boxes, bench
Plan to include jumping, rolling and balancing.

Mats
Revise your floorwork rolls and show me how you can link two or more rolls together.

Final Floor Activity
2 minutes

Balance; run and jump; balance.

Teaching notes and NC guidance
Development over 4 lessons

NC elements being emphasised:

a Exploring different means of rolling, jumping and balancing and adapting and refining these actions on the floor and on apparatus.
b Making appropriate decisions quickly and planning responses.
c Making judgements of performances and suggesting ways to improve.

Teaching Points

Anticipation, realisation and retrospect

If a good Physical Education lesson is 'like a good meal because you look forward to it, enjoy it, and remember it with great pleasure, and it has well-planned, satisfying variety', then this lesson should appeal. It has varied and lively, vigorous, exuberant running and jumping, contrasting with the more flowing, controlled rolling, contrasting with the still, firm balances.

Planning, performing and reflecting

Emphasise to the pupils the importance of planning before performance so that, for example in the apparatus sequence, they could tell you:

a their starting and finishing positions on floor and in body.
b the place where they run and jump into a turn on landing.
c which body part and piece of apparatus will be used for balance.
d where they will do their roll.

Emphasise, also, the value of reflecting immediately after their performance and trying to work out how to improve it next time. Often this reflecting and evaluating is inspired by the teacher, commenting in passing, or as a result of a demonstration given to the rest of the class and their follow-up comments, or as a result of seeing someone else's demonstration bringing out an interesting feature.

In NC terms, the pupils need to be 'put in the picture'; regarding the importance attaching to thoughtful planning and preparation as the basis for performance; to focused participating in the thoughtful way that enables reflection; and to reflecting and evaluating to bring in any changes or adaptations, as necessary, in their subsequent performances.

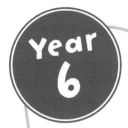

Year 6

Lesson Plan 4 • 30-35 minutes
December

Theme: *Body parts awareness and thinking beyond the action to how the hands, feet and larger body surfaces are working to carry, support, propel, grip and act generally.*

Floorwork
12—15 minutes

Legs

1 Take three walking steps, then do a hop. Step on to your non-hopping foot first.

2 Take three walking steps then do a long step. As before, start with the non take-off foot.

3 Now jump from one foot to both feet.

4 Can you join a hop, a step and a jump, starting with three walking steps?

Body

1 Hold a still, starting position on a part or parts of your body. Show me your different ways of moving your body on to a new supporting part or parts.

2 The sequence will be improved if you change levels.

3 Rolling, rocking, twisting, lowering, levering, jumping, swinging are among the many we have used.

Arms

1 Elbow balance. From a crouched position with feet apart, place hands on floor and under shoulders. Bend elbows slightly to place them inside and under knees. Tilt body forwards slowly, from feet on to hands, until toes come off the floor.

2 Show me a favourite way of taking weight on hands.

Apparatus Work
16—18 minutes

1 Using feet only, show actions you can use to take you along, over, across, around, through apparatus, without touching any.

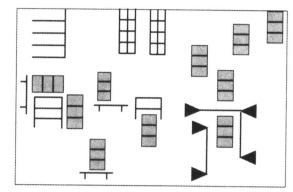

2 Using hands only, show me one touch only on apparatus where your touch can take you across, along or simply up into a balance.

3 At your apparatus starting places, can you practise, improve and remember the following?

Climbing frames
From a fixed position on one body part, can you travel by twisting, lowering, circling, pulling, levering strongly on to some other part?

Ropes
As you take off, swing and land, can you include varied actions at take-off and on landing?

Trestles
Use your arms strongly to bring you on to the apparatus. Plan ways to use them to grip, pull, support as you travel. And finally, can you make your hands important as you leave the apparatus?

Bench, box
Squat jump on to cross bench. Hands are shoulder width apart on the bench and feet are jumped on to bench, between hands. Jump off with a stretched or star jump. Squat jump on to end of long low box then use hands to help you along and from the box.

Mats
Revise your floorwork, transferring from body part to body part. Emphasise how you do the transfer.

Box, bench
Plan a sequence that includes vigorous jumps with soft landings, rolls and a slow body movement somewhere to contrast with the lively jumps.

Final Floor Activity
2 minutes

Sit with legs straight. Turn to front support. Jump feet to crouch. Spring up. Cartwheel.

Teaching notes and NC guidance
Development over 4 lessons

NC elements being emphasised:

a   Developing skill by exploring and making up activities.

b   Trying hard to consolidate their performances.

'What exactly is happening within our movements?' is what we are concentrating on in this lesson. This focus on our body parts and studying their exact actions takes us into the area of good quality and correct and safe techniques. 'Let your knees "give" on landing from a high jump'; 'Tuck your chin on to your chest (to safeguard head) as you roll forwards'; 'Keep your arms straight in your handstand'; 'Thumbs under the bar, fingers over, in climbing'; 'Thumbs forwards when doing a downward circle on a bar or pole'; 'Hands together when pulling up on a rope climb', etc.

When we train pupils to be good observers of movement to help them to make comments, judgements and even suggestions for improvement, we emphasise that the first two features they look out for are the actions being performed and the exact uses being made of the body parts involved. Body parts awareness leads to better body management and self-control. Such awareness comes from focusing on self and own movement. A greater repertoire and awareness of the huge range of body part uses is also developed by observing demonstrations and by the direct teaching of jumping and landing, climbing, rocking, rolling, lowering, tilting, twisting, springing, levering, overbalancing and leaning as methods of receiving, transferring and propelling our body weight.

Body parts awareness helps to improve control of our body shape, enhancing the appearance of the work, and making greater physical demands to make the whole body firm. Variety and contrast are two desirable features in a good Gymnastic Activities performance. Both are enhanced by an awareness of the many actions possible and the many ways in which body parts can function, in response to a challenge from the teacher. For example, stepping is only one of many 'travelling on feet' actions, but an awareness of the different actions and uses of body parts possible within stepping can produce great variety and contrast – on tiptoes, heels, inside and outside of foot; with straight, slightly bent, very bent knees; swinging leading leg forwards, to side, across you, behind before putting it down in front; in forward, sideways or backward directions.

Year 6

Lesson Plan 5 • 30-35 minutes
January

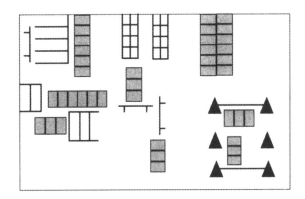

Theme: *Body shape awareness and a constant concern for good looking, poised movements.*

Floorwork
12–15 minutes

Legs

1 Walk smartly and briskly around the room as if you are on an important errand. Erect body with arms and legs swinging forwards well stretched.

2 Change to your best running where there is a look of 'lifting' in heels, arms, head and chest.

3 Now show me some running, jumping and landing where there is a clear body shape at all times.

Body

Stand, stretched on tiptoes; lower into a bridge on hands and feet; lower back on to seat and roll up to a stretched shoulder balance; twist bent legs over one shoulder to curled kneeling. Stand and repeat, and feel the many different body shapes you are holding or passing through.

Arms

1 In your handstanding or handwalking, experiment with legs stretched or bent, feet together or apart.

2 Balance is helped by very bent legs 'dangling' down low overhead and by legs making a straight line, one forwards, one held back, like a tightrope walker's pole.

Apparatus Work
16–18 minutes

1 Run freely all around the room, touching floor and mats only. When I call 'Stop!' show me a clear body shape on the nearest piece of apparatus. Stop!

2 Next time I stop you, can you match or contrast your body shape with that of someone near you. Stop!

3 **Climbing frames**

Can you travel to all parts of the frame, including going through spaces, by changing from a stretched to a curled body?

Ropes, mats, bench

a Revise your climbing, emphasising the 'one, two, hands together' to take hands up to a full stretch, followed by the full lift of both legs to their next gripping position.

b Swing and land on the mats with your body small and curled, then swing and land on the bench with your body almost straight.

Trestles

Can you use all the apparatus to show me held body shapes and shapes that you travel through?

Benches, mats

Run and jump high off the cross bench to show a different shape to the one who went before you. At the return long bench and mat, show me travelling actions where the body is straight, curled or wide.

Boxes, mats

Travel along the long box, demonstrating long body shapes. Travel across the cross, wide box, including at some point a wide body shape.

Mats

With a leader setting your group rhythm, practise again your floorwork sequence. Stretched on tiptoes; bridge on hands and feet roll to shoulder balance; twist to kneeling.

Final Floor Activity
2 minutes

Choose four neat body shapes, two on your left, and two on your right foot. Can you travel through each in turn on to the next?

Teaching notes and NC guidance
Development over 4 lessons

NC elements being emphasised:

a Emphasising changes of shape through physical actions.
b Adopting good posture and the appropriate use of the body.

Floorwork

Legs

1 Start by praising those who are standing well, head up, shoulders back, arms by sides, and weight slightly forwards on balls of feet, in a 'ready to go' position, and still, without fidgeting.

2 A quiet, lifting action works up from heels, through knees, arms, chest and head, all on the balls of the feet. Feeling is of 'up'.

Body

This directed sequence of four, varied, still, bridge-like shapes is led by the teacher and is a quick way to produce whole class activity. It shows a variety of supporting parts and body shapes. Pupils will move on to developing their own variations.

Arms

1 Because arms will always be stretched when inverted to ensure a safe, strong support for the whole body, variations of body shape will come from the leg positions, including, for example, one leg bent and one leg straight.

2 'Dangling legs' lower the centre of gravity to help balance.

Apparatus Work

1 A quick reaction and instant planning are needed to stop, go to nearest apparatus, and demonstrate a clear body shape. The teacher encourages balance on parts other than feet or feet and hands.

2 Pairs of adjacent performers now have to react quickly to present matching or (more difficult) contrasting body shapes. This activity deserves to be demonstrated, giving pleasure to several pairs and helpful ideas to everyone observing.

3 **Climbing frames**
There will be much feet only, then hands only travelling.

Ropes, mats, bench
a Hands together do the pulling, not the hand well above hand, often seen, where the bottom hand only works.
b Inspire a full swing by a strong up and back jump to give you a long, pendulum-like swing long enough to deliver you.

Trestles
A good challenge is 'Can you alternate still, held shapes with travelling shapes?'

Benches, mats
At cross bench, let one in front of you go, see the shape, then follow. At long bench, straight pulls, curled tight bunny jumps, wide, low cartwheels over, side to side.

Boxes, mats
Along with cartwheels, dive rolls, upward spring from crouch, pulls. Across with star jump off, low cartwheel across, hands on and feet wide astride on.

Mats
Group can be on opposite sides of mat, facing a space, with leader central.

Final Floor Activity

Go from left to right to left to right.

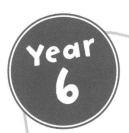

Lesson Plan 6 • 30-35 minutes
February

Theme: *Partner work to: (a) explore ways to work with another to create movements not possible when working alone; (b) gain a better understanding of own and others' talents and limitations.*

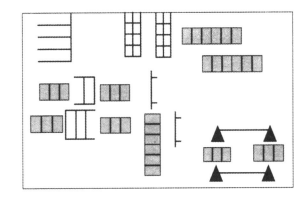

Floorwork
12–15 minutes

Legs

1   Follow your leader who varies the travelling by way of:
    a   using different parts of the foot
    b   varied directions
    c   varied shapes, tall, wide, small curled.

2   Other leader takes over and leads, varying the work by:
    a   changing speeds
    b   adding on unusual arm or leg 'gestures'.

Body

Take up a position near each other. Can you find different ways to grip each other and lean away from each other into a combined balance?

Arms

Partner 'A' takes up a strong position on hands and feet at a low level. Partner 'B' has to cross 'A' by taking weight on hands. ('A' has to make enough low, wide gaps to assist this.)

Apparatus Work
16–18 minutes

1   Follow your leader, using floor and mats only, walking, running and jumping when the available space makes these actions safe to use and appropriate.

2   One partner balancing, one partner giving a little support, hold a balance on a piece of apparatus, where the balance is perfectly firm, stretched and still. Change duties, still only giving minimum help to balance.

3   **Climbing frames**
    Start, side by side, at floor level. Can you travel upwards, sideways and down diagonally, together, showing good body shapes? Can you be aware of the shapes you are making as a pair?

    Ropes
    Rope each, starting facing each other. Can you make up a matching sequence which includes three examples of variety, such as body shapes used in travelling; directions used in travelling or on landing; methods of starting a swing.

    Trestles
    Start exactly opposite each other. Mirror each other's movements. Can you include a variety of travelling actions?

    Bench, upturned bench
    Follow your leader across bench on to mats where leader completes the first movement and waits for partner to copy and follow. On the return upturned bench can you both balance along, and keep some form of body contact?

    Boxes, mats
    Start at opposite ends of apparatus. Can you approach, meet, pass and finish in partner's starting place? On either box, can one partner hold a bridge for the other to negotiate?

    Mats
    Show your partner a favourite sequence of linked agilities. Your partner will observe carefully, then make one helpful suggestion for an improvement.

Final Floor Activity
2 minutes

With partner's support, show me a balance you could not do on your own. Each has a turn.

Teaching notes and NC guidance
Development over 4 lessons

NC elements being emphasised:

a Working safely, alone and with others.
b Practising, adapting, improving and repeating longer and increasingly complex sequences of movement.

Floorwork

Legs

1 Follow 2–3 metres behind to be able to see actions, body parts activity, shapes and directions easily. A routine of three activities is enough for one to plan and one to copy.

2 Second leader keeps same actions but expands them with a change of speed at one point, and a gesture, pointing with a body part.

Body

Lean away in identical or different standing, kneeling, sitting, side falling (on one hand and foot, side to floor), horizontal balance standing on one leg with trunk horizontal, crab, etc.

Arms

Partner crossing is looking for low arms, legs, back, best helped by long, low, wide star shape held by 'strong position' partner whose front, back or side can be towards the floor.

Apparatus Work

1 If the three actions are simple the pair can do them in unison, always looking for spaces and sometimes performing on the spot, one behind the other, when floor is suddenly crowded.

2 Minimum support, occasionally removing support for a moment as partner struggles to 'Hold it!'

3 **Climbing frames**
Travel up, then along to opposite side, and then diagonally back to start. A particular shape or shapes could be emphasised during each third.

Ropes
Plan: three or four actions; then uses of body parts concerned; then shapes; then changes of direction or levels.

Trestles
From matching start on signal of one of pair, approach, mount apparatus, leave apparatus, and travel to partner's starting place. Build up to performing in unison by keeping actions simple.

Bench, upturned bench
Contact along inverted bench by walking, one forwards, one back; both sideways; both forwards; one holds other who sits down on bench, etc.

Boxes, mats
At point of passing, one can be stationary, low to go over, high to go over.

Mats
'Agilities' mean activities mainly upended, supported by hands.

Final Floor Activity

For example, horizontal balance standing on one foot, with upper body leaning forwards as near horizontal as possible, and with both arms upstretched above head. Partner helps by placing a hand under one of partner's hands.

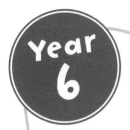

Lesson Plan 7 • 30-35 minutes
March

Theme: *Space awareness with an emphasis on making good and varied use of the floor and air space around us and the apparatus.*

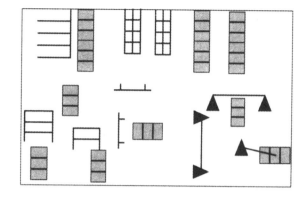

Floorwork
12—15 minutes

Legs

1 One half of the class run and jump, pushing arms and legs out strongly to take up as much air space as possible. The other half do quiet little jumps on the spot, taking as little air space as possible. The running and jumping, lively group must look for, then run into a new space each time.

2 Change over duties.

Body

1 Balance on your shoulders and explore your surrounding 'bubble' of space with your feet.

2 Lower to kneeling and explore your space 'bubble' with hands and upper body.

3 Are there any other starting positions from which you can reach out far into all parts of your space 'bubble'?

Arms

Place both hands firmly on the floor. Move in as many ways and to as many places as you can without moving hands.

Apparatus Work
16—18 minutes

Climbing frames, bench
Start at the bottom corner or bottom of bench. Zigzag your way to the top corner of the frame, and then come down diagonally to the opposite corner.

Rope, mats
a Can you climb from rope to rope, getting higher each time?

b Can you swing from mat to mat, or floor to mat, with legs at different levels? Can you include a direction change in the air or on landing?

Trestles, planks, pole, mats
a Travel, using all apparatus, with your body near to the apparatus.

b Travel, using all apparatus, with many parts of your body high above or stretched, well away from the apparatus.

Bench, upturned bench, trestle, mats
a Try some easy balances where you are low over your supporting parts.

b Try some balances where you are tall, wide, stretched and well above your supporting parts. Tall is harder to hold but better looking and more satisfying.

Boxes, mats
As you travel up to, on, along and from the apparatus, use as much air space as possible.

Mats
Link two rolls together where one is small, curled tight and not needing much space, and the other is bigger and needing more space.

Final Floor Activity
2 minutes

Practise an 'easy' jump in your own space, making a simple pattern or shape on the floor. Then travel about the whole space, repeating a big version of your pattern, and using much livelier actions.

Teaching notes and NC guidance
Development over 4 lessons

NC elements being emphasised:

a Emphasising changes of direction, level and use of own and shared space, through gymnastic actions.

b Exploring different means of jumping, balancing and taking weight on hands.

Floorwork

Legs

1 Often the air space, above, to front, rear and side of us, is not sufficiently considered in Gymnastic Activities. Here, it is the main consideration.

2 Often, we omit to perform on the spot, as we should do, when the floor ahead is suddenly crowded. Here, it is our main thought.

Body

1 Feet will split and reach to front, rear and to sides. With greater difficulty, feet can be held together as they reach out.

2 Arch to each side, to front, and to the rear which is the most difficult, particularly the return from being well arched back.

3 Standing with feet wide apart allows you to reach to all sides.

Arms

An arc of space, in a semi-circle, hands at centre; straight lines towards and back from hands; jumping feet to space between or outside of hands; bunny jumps into a low space above head; handstand into high space above head.

Apparatus Work

Climbing frames

Bench is hooked high on to a bar so that it is steeply inclined for travelling up, under or around.

Ropes, mats

a Emphasise transfer to a grip with both hands together, from a position with feet firmly crossed.

b Legs can swing hanging low; angled at a medium horizontal; or hooked high above hands on rope.

Trestles

a 'Near to' circling, sliding, crawling, hanging under with arms and legs wrapped around.

b 'High balance' on one foot, on tiptoes, sitting astride, high kneeling, upended on shoulders.

Bench, upturned bench, trestle, mats

a 'Low balances' on all fours, on one hand and one foot, sitting, side towards on one hand and one foot.

b 'Tall balances' on tiptoes, one foot, shoulders.

Boxes, mats

High, wide shaped jumps up and from apparatus.

Mats

The small, slow forward roll can be from a starting, crouch position, reaching down to just in front of feet. The bigger roll can be longer and quicker with a dive to lift you momentarily off the floor, over an imaginary obstacle.

Final Floor Activity

The floor patterns that lend themselves to work on the spot, then work in the whole room space, include circles, triangles, straight line corridors, figures of eight.

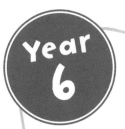

Lesson Plan 8 • 30–35 minutes
April

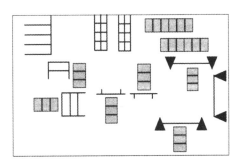

Theme: *Good use of effort to achieve controlled performance: we are concerned with the degree of force being applied, and the amount of speed being used.*

Floorwork
12–15 minutes

Legs

1   Run with a relaxed, 'easy' action that feels effortless.

2   Now, change between slow running when you have little space, and quick running when there is plenty of room.

3   Can you link together an easy, soft jump on the spot; slow running; then a quick run into an explosive, upward jump?

Body

1   From a still standing position, lower to sitting and rock smoothly back on to shoulders and hands. Balance still, then rock back to standing, building up speed for a strong spring up on to feet.

2   A variation could be a start, balanced on one foot with the other leg and both arms stretched well forwards, before your very slow lower to sitting. Your speedy return, if powerful enough, could take you up on to one foot only, again.

Arms

1   Can you hold a handstand for three seconds, using spread fingers strongly to control you?

2   In how many ways can you come down, softly, under control?

3   If you prefer, show me your longest, slowest ever cartwheel.

Apparatus Work
16–18 minutes

Climbing frames

Travel in many directions, using two hands then two feet. Can you include moments when your whole body is being supported by your hands?

Boxes, mats

a   Can you plan a sequence to include favourite activities across box and along long return box? Include good gymnastic links between the lines.

b   Make your work even more interesting by showing a contrast in speed or force applied.

Trestles

a   Start and finish on the floor. Show ways to mount on to the apparatus, using arms or legs strongly.

b   Use your hands strongly to return you gently to the floor.

Mats

a   Revise cartwheel, emphasising firm, stretched body position and four long counts of hand, hand, foot, foot.

b   At return mats, practise a forward roll to standing with one foot behind the other. Swivel body around to side of rear foot and finish with a backward roll.

Ropes

Revise leading-up stages to rope climbing as appropriate for each child.

a   Swing freely on rope, practising hands together grip.

b   Swing from sitting on a chair to let you secure a strong, crossed foot grip.

c   Swing from standing and try to take one hand off to prove a strong foot grip.

d   Climb. Hand; hand; hands together; feet up.

Benches, mats

From a position on the cross bench, can you transfer slowly to the mats, making your hands important? At the return cross bench, show a lively, contrasting movement where your legs are important.

Final Floor Activity
2 minutes

Walk, run, jump and land where feet land one after the other, gradually slowing to a still finish.

Teaching notes and NC guidance
Development over 4 lessons

NC elements being emphasised:

a Emphasising changes of speed and effort through gymnastic actions.

b Making appropriate decisions quickly and planning their responses.

Floorwork

Legs

1 When we apply effort and body tension, we can 'feel' how we are moving. We want to feel so easy that we could keep on going.

2 Slow running, including running on the spot if necessary to avoid others, is accompanied by a lowering of arms and heels and an upright body. In quicker running, we incline forwards more and lift heels, knees and arms more for the rapid striding.

3 Gentle effort; slow motion; accelerating motion into maximum effect are all represented and asked for in this sequence.

Body

1 The build up of speed to rock you back from shoulder balance to standing is helped by a vigorous, strong leg swing.

2 Variety in return from shoulder balance includes a slight change of direction, and coming up on to one foot or to feet crossed.

Arms

1 A good hand balance starts with just the right amount of arms and leg swing to take you up. We have to practise and remember how it feels when it is just right.

2 The soft, gentle return to standing contrasts with the strong firm push up.

3 Slow work on hands, all looking neat and well controlled, is our aim – plus the excellent physical demands being made on arms and shoulder muscles.

Apparatus Work

Climbing frames

Particularly when supported by hands only, keep both thumbs gripping under the bars, fingers over, for a safe, strong hold.

Boxes, mats

a Make work non-stop by including jumps, rolls or cartwheels between the two lines, rather than just walking between.

b Work on hands and rolls can be slow. Jumps can be dynamic.

Trestles

a Strong hand action is needed to grip and hang below; or push to lift up and on; to grip sides and pull along; to circle around and on to; to twist across or on.

b Leave, using hands as you circle around pole; as you roll from sitting or kneeling; as you bunny jump off; as you twist from.

Mats

a Even if cartwheel is diagonal to floor, rather than vertical, a firm, stretched body can be demonstrated.

b Shoulder above crossed behind foot swings around into the turn.

Ropes

Emphasise hands together grip when pulling both feet up to their next, crossed feet together grip.

Benches

Slow, strong hands contrast with sudden, explosive legs.

Final Floor Activity

Accelerate into the jump and try to decelerate on landing, to a still finish position.

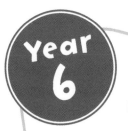
Lesson Plan 9 • 30-35 minutes
May

Theme: *Revision and direct teaching of simple, traditional gymnastic skills.*

Floorwork
12–15 minutes

Legs

1 Using three running steps, only, each time, run and jump up with a stretch, a wide star and a tuck, moving on a triangular pathway.

2 Stand. Do a jump up and a half-turn, swinging one arm across to create the turn. Right arm swings when jumping up and turning to the left.

Body

1 Stand, balanced on one leg, with upper body inclined well forwards, arms upstretched, and other leg stretched well back.

2 Lower back and down to balance, sitting with head up, legs straight and together, and arms stretched sideways for balance. (Seat only on floor.)

3 Rock back to shoulder balance with legs straight and together. Hands can either support hips at rear, or press hard down on floor.

4 Swing back up to standing and repeat.

Arms

We have been doing our handstands and cartwheels from a standing position. Try to co-ordinate a two or three step run into either or both. The extra momentum will help you to invert more easily and quickly.

Apparatus Work
16–18 minutes

Mats
Try to link together two of your favourite agilities.

Climbing frames
Rotary descent from top bars. Sit at top, with hands crossed on bar at face height. One hand grips with knuckles towards you, the other grips with knuckles away from you. Lower your body by

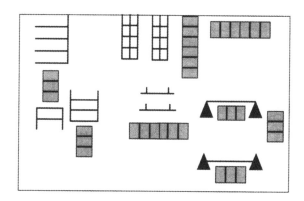

twisting the shoulder of the near hand (knuckles towards you) backwards. You will lower, turning, to the bar below.

Ropes
a Circle backwards, gripping two ropes at shoulder height, by lifting both legs up and over head.
b Reverse hanging on two ropes. Hands at shoulder height, lift legs up and off floor to stretch them up towards ceiling, or hook one leg around each rope.

Upturned benches, mats
a On parallel benches, balance walk with some contact with a partner.
b On mats, practise going from elbow balance into a bent leg headstand.

Boxes, mats
Cat spring on to end of long box top. Either cat spring, roll, cartwheel or vault off the other end. At cross box, face vault or gate vault over. 'Face vault' is like a high bunny jump and you twist over, facing box top, all the way. 'Gate vault' has hands facing forwards, legs lift straight to one side as they come around and down, with hand on swinging side lifting off.

Trestles
Circle up and down on metal pole. Roll from planks on to mats. Upward jumps with half-turns from planks.

Final Floor Activity
2 minutes

Start at the back of the room. Run forwards to opposite end, and do your three starting jumps before reaching the other end. Turn, and we will all go back again.

Teaching notes and NC guidance
Development over 4 lessons

NC elements being emphasised:

a Responding readily to instructions.

b Sustaining energetic activity and working vigorously to develop suppleness and strength and to exercise the heart and lungs strongly.

Floorwork

Legs

1 'Good things happen in threes' and a triangle of jumps brings you back to own starting place. Runs are short, about 3 metres. Jumps are the main thing.

2 Four jumps on the spot facing forwards can be followed by two, each of which includes a quarter turn. Four more on the spot, then two with a quarter turn to bring you back to start.

Body

1 First position is called horizontal balance standing.

2 The sitting balance has the body tilted back slightly with a strong effort to keep back, arms and legs all stretched.

3 Feet with stretched ankles should be above hips, which should be above shoulders, all in a line, balanced on shoulders.

4 Legs swing strongly, then bend under you to take you standing.

Arms

This walk and skip with one leg and both arms swinging up together can lead into a handstand practice on the floor, against a wall, or against the supporting teacher.

Apparatus Work

Mats

You can show your work to a partner who will tell you what he or she liked, and one way in which you can improve. Partner might ask for clearer shapes and neater, still start and finish.

Climbing frames

Strong arm and shoulder exercise with strong abdominal exercise as you lift your legs to twist down each time. Momentarily, all body weight is supported by arms but tummy muscles work hard to lift seat and legs clear of bar.

Ropes

a Shoulder height grip important to ensure feet come down to floor again, and not left dangling in mid-air. Bent, short lever legs easier to lift into circle than straight legs.

b Let them choose to hook feet around ropes, or try to hold them straight together, away from ropes.

Upturned benches, mats

a Walk facing each other; side by side; facing opposite directions, hand in hand, hand on shoulder.

b Legs are bent in elbow balance, from which you lower slowly on to forehead and hands.

Boxes, mats

Face vault much easier than gate vault.

Trestles

The attractive variety from rolls, circles and jumps is worth demonstrating, particularly if virtually non-stop with a good group, sharing, thinking ahead and never queuing.

Final Floor Activity

Run and jump stretched, run and jump wide, run and jump tucked.

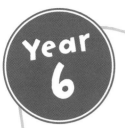

Lesson Plan 10 • 30-35 minutes
June

Theme: *Partner work with emphasis on matching and contrasting movements. Observing, copying or contrasting a partner's movement develops one's powers of observation and an awareness of the elements of movement.*

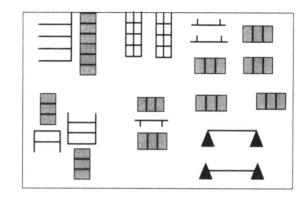

Floorwork
12–15 minutes

Legs

One behind other, about 1–2 metres apart, the leader travels on feet and then stops. At each restart, a slight change of direction, body shape or speed is introduced in the next travel and stop and the actions can change.

Body

With other partner now as leader, the couples face each other. Start in a half-kneeling position on one lower leg and the opposite hand. In your three or four balance sequence, use a variety of supporting parts and interesting linking movements.

Arms

'A' makes various bridges, supported strongly on hands and feet. 'B' travels under, over, through or around 'A' using hands and feet only as supports. Change over duties.

Apparatus Work
16–18 minutes

Climbing frames
Can you show me ways of travelling over, under and around each other?

Upturned benches
a   On the parallel upturned benches, keep some contact with your partner as you balance forwards, sideways or backwards.
b   Support your partner in a bent leg headstand.

Ropes
Using ropes, floor and mats, can you plan a matching sequence, done together?

Trestles
Start at opposite sides or ends of the apparatus. Approach, meet, negotiate each other, finish in partner's starting place.

Cross bench, mats
Starting at opposite sides, can you build up to a matching approach, flight and landing?

Boxes, mats
Watch your partner's sequence which includes a jump, a roll and taking all the weight on hands at some point. While your partner practises, improves and remembers his or her sequence, can you, the observer, create a contrasting sequence? (For example, different shape in the jump; a roll in the opposite direction, or at a different speed; weight on hands with a different leg shape or action.)

Final Floor Activity
2 minutes

Side by side, jump up on the spot; run three steps into a high matching jump and identical landing; jump up into a half-turn and repeat.

Teaching notes and NC guidance
Development over 4 lessons

NC elements being emphasised:

a Working safely, alone and with others.

b Developing skill by exploring and making up activities and by expressing themselves imaginatively.

Floorwork

Legs

Because there has to be a travel and a stop, the following, copying partner can stand still, observing and remembering the action, and then catch up with the leader each time. The challenge for the observer is to recognise the nature of the 'slight change' each time, and, of course, for the leader to put one in. If using demonstrations here, ask the observers 'What changes did you see?'

Body

The new leader is asked for a variety of supporting parts and slow, smooth linking movements. Emphasise that it is a balance sequence, requiring difficulty in holding the balance on a small or unusual body part or parts. Good pairs, mirroring each other in exact unison, deserve to be presented for a demonstration.

Arms

Both partners are to be supported on hands and feet, with the stationary partner sufficiently high and arched to leave room for travelling by the partner. 'A' can bridge with front, back or side to the floor and change bridges to give partner a new challenge to negotiate.

Apparatus Work

Climbing frames

One partner can stay and work in centre four spaces while other travels across, around, under or over him or her.

Upturned benches

a They can face opposite ways to travel; touch each other with different body parts (hands, elbows, hand to shoulder, hands to shoulders), and show same or contrasting shapes.

b Supporting partner kneels in front of partner, lifting hips and back against own chest as partner walks in and lifts to headstand.

Ropes

Aim for a matching stationary start; then a matching side by side travel (e.g. swing and forward roll, or swing and cartwheel); then a still, matching finish.

Trestles

At the point of 'negotiation', one can be stationary while the other travels under, over or past him or her.

Cross bench, mats

A starting signal by one partner can be a little lifting of heels by one, signifying 'Now!' (Let's go!)

Boxes, mats

The elements to consider in planning for contrast are: shape; direction; speed; and different uses of body parts. (For example, a diving, stretched roll forwards, done vigorously to contrast with a sideways, tightly curled roll, slowly and easily.) This difficult challenge needs good observation and planning.

Final Floor Activity

Couples work, side by side, or one slightly ahead, back and forwards, in a narrow corridor, only 3–4 metres in length. The starting signal can be a slight knees bend by the leader, just before the jump.

Year 6

Lesson Plan 11 • 30-35 minutes
July

Theme: *Sequences, through which the children work harder for longer, expressing vigour, skilfulness, understanding and, it is hoped, enthusiasm, enjoyment and satisfaction.*

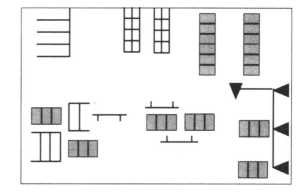

Floorwork
12–15 minutes

Legs

Show me a sequence where you work on the spot to start with, then travel to a new space of your own. Can you plan to include more than one kind of leg action, and examples of both gentle and vigorous movements?

Body

Including a lunge among your stretches, can you travel using stretching and curling movements? Working at different levels, using different supporting parts, will provide interesting variety.

Arms

Travel, using feet and hands where you emphasise the varied pattern of possible foot and hand movements. They can move alternately; left side only; right side only; apart; together; or run and cartwheel or handstand, etc.

Apparatus Work
16–18 minutes

Climbing frames

a Using floor and apparatus, can you balance, travel, balance using a variety of supporting parts in your balances?

b Can you plan to include being vertical, horizontal and upended?

Ropes

a In your climbing emphasise the full stretch after the three count hand shift, and the full curl after the high leg lift.

b Show me a sequence of three swings that include a change of direction, speed and body shape.

Inverted benches, mats

In your balancing along the benches, travel at different levels and include a change of direction somewhere. At the mats, revise elbow balance and/or bent leg headstand.

Boxes, mats

Can you include a rolling action along the low long box and mats? Show me a vaulting action with shoulders over hands on the return cross box. Try to plan for a long flowing sequence with neat links between the lines.

Trestles, planks, pole, mats

Can you travel, using all the apparatus, with feet leading or following on, under, across, around and along the apparatus?

Mats

Show me a balance, roll, balance sequence where you include at least one upended balance and a change of direction somewhere. At the return mats can you do a forward roll followed by a dive forward roll (i.e. whole of body in air at one point)?

Final Floor Activity
2 minutes

Using legs only, make up a sequence of walking, running and jumping which includes varied actions in flight. For example: hurdling; jacknife; scissors; tuck; rolling one leg over the other.

Teaching notes and NC guidance
Development over 4 lessons

NC elements being emphasised:

a   Making appropriate decisions quickly and planning their responses.
b   Practising, adapting, improving and repeating longer and increasingly complex sequences of movement.
c   Making judgements and suggesting ways to improve.

Teaching Points

These sequences and performances show the level of skilfulness, knowledge, understanding and attitudes that have developed during the four years of the Gymnastic Activities course.

Skills

1   The ability to plan, perform, remember and refine a series of movements into a pleasing, varied sequence which answers the task.

2   The ability to demonstrate control, poise, vigour and versatility in sequences which make full use of all 'movement' elements.

Knowledge and understanding

1   Awareness of the 'movement' elements that influence quality and aesthetic appeal in gymnastic performances – variety, contrast, repetition, body tension and clarity of shape.

2   Understanding how to apply these movement elements to the parts of a sequence to make the performance more demanding, and more interesting and satisfying to performer and spectator.

Desirable class attitudes

'What you don't use, you lose. We, the class, have continually been taught and encouraged to develop and make full use of our strength, stamina, suppleness and versatility. These lessons have been good fun, exciting and good for us. We believe that they have made us very fit because of the way the whole body is being exercised so strongly. We also believe that you look and feel better if you exercise regularly.

   Working with others; learning with them and from them; giving and receiving demonstrations; and hearing their friendly, encouraging comments have all made these lessons particularly sociable and friendly and brought our class together in a special way. Our teacher has said that we will be remembered for our whole-hearted, co-operative, enthusiastic responses, neat, well controlled, versatile, high quality work, and our capacity for working hard to achieve success.'

Dance

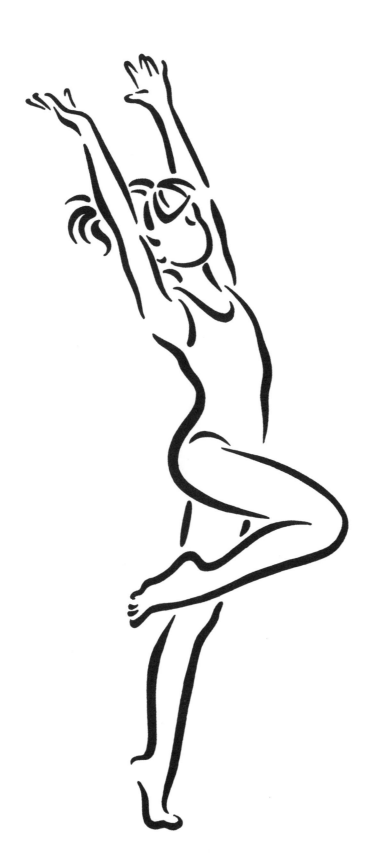

The Aims of Dance

Education has been described as the 'structuring of experiences in such a way as to bring about an increase in human capacity.' Dance aims to increase human capacity under the following headings:

1 **Physical development**. We focus on body action to develop skilful, well-controlled, versatile movement. We want our pupils to move well, looking poised and confident. The vigorous actions in dance also promote healthy physical development, fitness and strength.

2 **Knowledge and understanding**. Pupils learn and understand through the combination of physical activity (with its doing, feeling and experiencing of movement) and the mental processes of decision-making, as they plan, refine, evaluate and then plan again for improvement.

3 **Enjoyment**. Dance is fun and an interesting, sociable, enjoyable physical activity. In addition to the perspiration and deep breathing which the vigorous physical activity inspires, there should be smiling faces expressing enjoyment. When asked why they like something, pupils' first answer is usually 'It's fun!' It is hoped that enjoyable, sociable and physical activity experienced regularly at school in dance and other physical education lessons, can have an influence on pupils' eventual choice of lifestyle, long after they have left school. We want them to understand that regular physical activity makes you look and feel better, and helps to make you feel relaxed, calm and fit.

4 **Confidence and self-esteem**. Particularly at primary school, a good physical education that recognises and praises achievement can enhance an individual's regard for him or herself, and help to improve confidence and self-esteem. Dance lessons are extremely visual and offer many opportunities to see improvement, success and creativity; demonstrating these admirable achievements to others; and helping pupils feel good about themselves.

5 **Social development**. Friendly, co-operative social relationships are part of most dance lessons. Achievement, particularly in the 'dance climax' part of the lesson, is usually shared with a partner or a small group. Pupils also share space sensibly with others; take turns at working; demonstrate to, and watch demonstrations by, others; and make appreciative, helpful comments to demonstrators and partners.

6 **Creativity**. It has been said that 'if you have never created something, you have never experienced satisfaction.' Dance is a most satisfying activity, regularly challenging pupils to plan and present something original. Opportunities abound for an appreciative teacher to say 'Thank you for your demonstration and your own, original way of doing the movements.'

7 **Expression and communication**. In dance we communicate through the expression in movement of the feelings or the action. We use, for example, stamping feet to express anger; we skip, punch the air or clap hands to show happiness; we swagger, head held high, to express self-assurance. Similarly, we create simple characters and stories by expressing them through movements associated with them. The old or young; machine or leaves; puppet, animal or circus clown, can all be expressed through their particular way of moving.

8 **Artistic and aesthetic appreciation**. Gaining knowledge and understanding of the quality-enhancing elements of movement is a particular aim of dance. Such understanding of quality, variety and contrast in the use of body action, shape, direction, size, speed and force, is a major contributor to appreciation of good movement. We want our pupils to understand what is good about good movement.

Stimuli as Starting Points With Which to Inspire Dance Action

Stimuli are used to gain the interest of the class, provide a focus for their attention, get them into the action quickly, and inspire in them a desire for movement.

A dance stimulus is something you:

○ **enjoy doing**, such as natural actions. Pupils will immediately start to walk, run, jump, skip, hop, bounce or gallop, whether accompanied by music, percussion, following the teacher/leader, or responding to an enthusiastic teacher calling out the actions.

○ **can hear**. Sounds that stimulate movement include:

  a medium to quick tempo music, including folk dance music

  b percussion instruments – tambourine, drum, cymbal, clappers

  c body contact sounds – clapping hands, stamping feet, slapping body, clicking fingers

  d rhythmically chanted phrases, words, place names or actions which can be shortened or elongated to inspire and accompany actions

  e vocal sounds to accompany actions, on the spot and travelling as in 'toom, toom, toom' marching; 'boomp, boomp, boomp' bouncing; and 'tick, tock, tick, tock' slow stepping

  f action songs, chanted rhymes and nursery rhymes.

○ **can see or imagine**. Objects like a leaf, branch, balloon, ball, bubble, puppet, rag doll, firework, can all be used to suggest movement ideas to children. Use of imagery and imagination helps to communicate what we are trying to express more clearly. 'Can you creep softly and slowly, as if you did not want to be heard, coming home late?'

○ **have seen on a visit, on television, or in a photograph**. Of particular interest to pupils are:

  a zoo animals – penguins. elephants, dolphins, monkeys

  b circus performers – jugglers, clowns, trapeze artists, acrobats, tightrope walkers

  c seaside play – swimming, paddling, making sandcastles, plus movements of the waves

  d children's playground activities – climbing, swinging, sea-saw, throwing and catching, skipping, circling on a roundabout.

○ **experience seasonally** – spring and growth, summer holidays, autumn and harvest, winter snow and frost, Guy Fawkes' Night, Halloween, Christmas toys, circus and pantomime, Easter eggs.

○ **consider newsworthy or of human interest** – Olympic Games, extremes of weather, newly arrived pupils, hobbies, family, friendship, approaching holidays.

Whatever the starting point, the teacher must convert it into the language of movement. Children cannot 'be' leaves, but they can 'Travel on tip toes with light, floating movements, tilting and turning slowly.' They cannot 'be' clowns, but they can 'Do a funny walk on heels, spin round with one leg high, fall down slowly, bounce up and repeat.' They cannot 'be' machines, but they can 'Try pushing down actions, like corks into bottles, on the spot, turning or moving along, as on an assembly line.'

The Creative Dance Lesson Plan

Warming up Activities which start the lesson are important because they can create an attentive, co-operative, industrious and thoughtful start to the lesson, put the class in the mood for dance, and encourage them to move with good body poise and tension, sharing the floor unselfishly. The activities need to be simple enough to get the whole class working, almost immediately, often by following the teacher who, ideally, is a stimulating **'purveyor of action'** enthusiastically leading the whole class, often by example, into wholehearted participation in simple activities which need little explanation. Some form of travelling, using the feet, is often the warming-up activity, with a specific way of moving being asked for. It might be to show better use of space, greater variety, greater control, good poise and body tension, or simply an enthusiastic use of all the body parts to warm up.

The Movement Skills Training middle part of the lesson is used to teach and develop the movement skills and patterns that are to be used in the new dance. Here, the teacher is an **educator**, informing, challenging, questioning, using demonstrations and sometimes direct teaching.

a Kneel down and curl to your smallest shape. Show me how you can start to grow, very slowly. Are you starting with your back, head, shoulders, elbows or arms? Show me clearly how you rise to a full, wide stretch position.

b If gesturing is like speaking with your body's movement, how might your body gesture say 'I am angry'? Stamp feet, clench fists, punch the air, jump up and down heavily.

c How are bubbles (made by teacher and pupils) moving? Where are they going? Floating gently, gliding smoothly, soaring from low to higher, sinking slowly.

The creating and performing Dance Climax of the lesson is the most important part and must not be missed out or rushed. If necessary, earlier parts of the lesson should be reduced. Here the teacher is a **coach**, helping and guiding the pupils as they work at their creation, moving round to all parts of the room to advise, encourage, enthuse, praise and, eventually, demonstrate.

a Slowly, start to grow and show me which parts are leading as you rise to your full, wide flower shape in our 'Spring Dance'. You might even twist your flower shape to look at the sun.

b Find a partner for our 'Gestures' dance and decide who is asking a favour by gesturing with body actions to say 'Please! I'm desperate! I need it! I must have it!' The other partner's body actions are saying 'Never! You must be joking! Go away!' When we look at demonstrations later, we will decide who the most expressive winners are.

c For our 'Bubbles dance', I will say the four actions that are to be practised – floating gently, gliding smoothly, soaring, sinking slowly, and you will show me how you have planned to dance them.

Depending on its complexity, a dance lesson will be repeated three or four times to allow sufficient time for repetition, practice and improvement to take place, and a satisfactory performance to be achieved and presented.

It has been said that 'dance is all about making, remembering and repeating patterns.' Whether we are performing a created dance or an existing folk dance, there will still be a still start and finish, and an arrangement of repeated parts within.

The Traditional Folk Dance Lesson Plan – 30 minutes

Warming-up activities – 5 minutes

These varied steps can relate to the new figures to be taught, or they can be travelling steps or steps on the spot of any kind, to stimulate quick, easy enjoyable action to put the class in the mood for dance. The warm-up can be done alone or with a partner. As well as inspiring action, the teacher establishes high standards of neat footwork and good, safe, unselfish sharing of space. For example, 'Skip by yourself, to visit all parts of the room, keeping in time with the music.' 'When drum sounds twice, join hands with the nearest person and dance together.' 'When drum sounds once, dance by yourself again.'

Teach figures of new dance – 14 minutes

Teaching is easier in a big circle formation where everyone can see and copy the teacher. Often, all can perform the whole dance together, slowly and carefully, figure by figure, practising it to the teacher's voice, then doing it at the correct speed. The teacher's non-stop vocal accompaniment, along with the actions, serves to remind the class of the actions and keeps them moving at the correct speed. For example, 'Everyone ready... Skip to the centre, 2, 3, turn on 4; back to places, 2, 3, arrive on 4. Boys to centre, 2, 3, turn on 4; back to places, 2, 3, there on 4. Girls to centre, 2, 3, turn on 4; back to places, 2, 3, hands joined on 4. All circle left, 2, 3, 4, 5, 6, back the other way; circle right, 2, 3, 4, 5, 6, ready to start again.'

Teaching in sets of two, three, four or more couples is more difficult because the sets are separate, with someone's back to the teacher. Each leading couple in turn will be taken slowly through the figures, then walking, then dancing to the music or the teacher's vocal accompaniment.

Teach the new dance – 7 minutes

Ideally, the new dance will be performed without stopping, helped by early reminders to the next dancers from the teacher's continuous vocal accompaniment. It is sometimes necessary to stop the music after each dancing couple has completed the dance, because of problems experienced by some of the dancers. The new couples are put in position, the music is re-started, and they do the dance once again.

Revise a favourite dance – 4 minutes

This last dance, often chosen by pupils, should be a contrast to the lesson's new dance, for variety. A lively circle dance, with all dancing non-stop, can be contrasted with a set dance where only one or two of the four couples are dancing at a time.

Teaching Dance With 'Pace'

High on the list of accolades for an excellent dance lesson is the comment that 'it had excellent pace' and moved along, almost non-stop, from start to finish. Lesson pace is determined by the way that each of the several skills making up the whole lesson is taught. For example:

1   **Quickly into action**. Using few words, explain the skill clearly and challenge the class to begin. 'Show me your best stepping, in time with the music. Begin!' This near-instant start is helped if the teacher joins in and works enthusiastically with them.

2   **Emphasise the main teaching points, one at a time, while class is working**. The class all need to be working quietly if the teacher is to be heard. 'Visit all parts of the room – sides, ends and corners, as well as the middle.' 'Travel along straight lines, never following anyone.' (Primary school pupils always travel in a big anti-clockwise circle, all following one another, unless taught otherwise.)

3   **Identify and praise good work while the class is working**. The class teacher does not say 'well done' without being specific and explaining what is praiseworthy. Comments are heard by all and remind the class of key points. 'Well done, Kate. Your tip toe stepping is lively and neat.' 'Ahmed, you keep finding good spaces to travel through. Well done.'

4   **Teach for individual improvement, while the class is working**. 'Thomas, swing arms and legs with more determination, please.' 'Lucy, use your eyes each time you change direction to see where the best space is.'

5   **Use a demonstration, briefly**, to show good quality, or a good example of what is expected and worth copying. 'Stop, please, and watch Chloe, Michael, James and Fatima step out firmly with neat, quiet footwork, never following anyone.' 'Stop and watch how Rachel is mixing bent, straight and swinging leg actions for variety.'

6   **Very occasionally, to avoid using too much activity time, a short demonstration is followed by comments from observers**. 'Half of the class will watch the other half. Look out for and tell me whose stepping is neat, lively and always well spaced. Tell me if someone impresses you for any other reason.' The class watch for about 12 seconds and three or four comments are listened to. For example: 'Leroy is mixing tiny steps with big ones.' 'Maisie is stepping with feet passing each other, then with feet wide apart.' Halves of the class change over and repeat the demonstrations with comments.

7   **Thanks are given to all the performers and to those who made helpful, friendly comments**. Further practice takes place with reminders of the good things seen and commented on.

A Pattern for Looking at and Developing Dance Movement

To avoid confusing him or herself and the class, the teacher will be thinking about, looking for and talking about one element within dance at a time. If, in the early stages of a lesson's development, the teacher is only looking for the actions and how the body parts concerned are performing them, there is some hope for progress and improvement. If, on the other hand, the teacher is exhorting the class to think about 'your spacing, actions, shape, speed – and what about some direction changes?', all at the same time, then confusion will be the only outcome.

Stage 1 The Body

What is the pupil doing?

1 **Actions** travelling, jumping, turning, rolling, balancing, gesturing, rising, falling, etc..

2 **Body parts important** legs, feet, hands, shoulders, head, etc..

3 **Body shape** stretched, curled, wide. twisted, arched.

Stage 2 The Space

Where is the pupil doing it?

1 **Directions** forwards, backwards, sideways.

2 **Level** high, medium, low.

3 **Size** own, little, personal space; whole room, large general space shared with others.

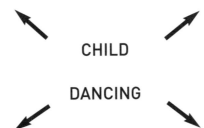

CHILD

DANCING

Stage 3 The Quality

How is the pupil doing it?

1 **Weight or effort** firm, gentle, vigorous, light, heavy.

2 **Time or speed** sudden, fast, slow, speeding up, slowing down, explosive.

Stage 4 The Relationships

With whom is the pupil doing it?

1 **Alone** but always conscious of sharing space with others.

2 **Teacher** near, following, mirroring, in circle with, away from, towards.

3 **Partner** leading, following, meeting, parting, mirroring, copying, making contact with.

4 **Group** circle, part of class for a demonstration

Headings When Considering a Pupil's Achievement and Progress Through Dance

Physical fitness

Strong, often prolonged physical activity, inspired by vigorous leg action, helps to promote normal, healthy growth and physical development. Lively leg action in dance also stimulates strong heart and lungs activity, leading to improved stamina.

Physical skill and versatility

Body management and self-control, called for in challenging situations, develops skill in natural actions such as travelling, jumping and landing, balancing, rolling, turning, rising and falling. When body management and self-control are good, there is an impression of poised, confident, versatile, safe movement.

Feeling valued and self-confident

Using their imagination, being creative, planning something original, and then sharing it with others, can develop and improve pupils' self confidence and self-esteem, particularly when the teacher and the class warmly and enthusiastically express their appreciation for the achievement. We want our dancers, eventually, to exude confidence and enthusiasm.

Expressing themselves

Using the body as an instrument of expression, and another way to communicate, pupils can express emotions, inner feelings, moods, convey ideas, and even create simple characters and stories. For many, this is a totally different, potentially eloquent outlet for expressing feeling as they stamp the work with their own personality.

Learning to develop friendly, co-operative, working relationships with others

Dance is the most sociable of physical education's activities. Working in pairs and groups; sharing space; taking turns; demonstrating and being demonstrated to; and appreciating and being appreciated by others, encourages desirable, enjoyable, co-operative social relationships.

Believing in the value of participation in physical activity

We want pupils to look and feel better after exercise, and believe that physical activity is enjoyable, and an essential antidote to the increasingly sedentary, inactive lifestyle of many people.

Becoming more competent, knowledgeable performers and spectators

Dance education develops an appreciation of the aesthetic and expressive elements within dance – variety and contrast in actions, shape, direction and level, speed, and degree of force.

National Curriculum Requirements for Dance – Key Stage 2: the Main Features

Programme of study Pupils should be taught to:

a   create and perform dances using a range of movement patterns, including those from different times and cultures

b   respond to a range of stimuli and accompaniment.

Attainment targets Pupils should be able to demonstrate that they can:

a   link skills, techniques and ideas and apply them accurately and appropriately, showing precision, control and fluency

b   compare and comment on skills, techniques and ideas used in others' work, and use this understanding to improve their own performance by modifying and refining skills and techniques.

Main NC headings when considering progression and expectation

Planning – This provides the focus and the concentrated thinking necessary for an accurate performance. Where standards of planning are satisfactory, there is evidence of:

a   the ability to think ahead, visualising what you want to achieve

b   good decision-making, selecting the most appropriate choices

c   a good understanding of what was asked for

d   an understanding of the elements of quality, variety and contrast

e   an unselfish willingness to listen to others' views and adapt own performance correspondingly.

Performing and improving performance – This is always the most important feature of a lesson. We are fortunate that the visual nature of Physical Education enables pupils' achievement to be easily seen, shared and judged. Where standards in performing are satisfactory, there is evidence of:

a   successful, safe outcomes

b   neat, accurate, 'correct' performances

c   consistency, and the ability to repeat and remember

d   economy of effort and making everything look 'easy'

e   adaptability, making sudden adjustments as required.

Linking actions – With a view to getting pupils working harder for longer, which is a main aim for Physical Education teaching, encourage them to pursue near-continuous, vigorous and enjoyable action, expressed ideally in deep breathing, perspiration and smiling faces.

Reflecting and evaluating – These factors are important because they help both the performers and the observers with their further planning, preparation, adapting and improving. Where standards are satisfactory, there is evidence of:

a   recognition of key features and keen and accurate observation

b   awareness of accuracy of work

c   helpful suggestions for improvement

d   good self-evaluation and acting upon these reflections

e   sensitive concern for another's feelings, and a good choice of words regarding another's work.

Year 6 Dance Programme

Pupils should be able to:

Autumn	Spring	Summer
1 Perform dance steps with skill, accuracy and increased poise.	1 Repeat sequences with increasing control and accuracy.	1 Move with increased poise, control and co-ordination.
2 Perform more complex patterns of movement, neatly linked, with interesting use of shapes, speed, directions and effort.	2 Compose and control movements by varying shape, direction, speed and effort.	2 Be able to improve, repeat and remember a dance, focusing on one main movement feature at a time.
3 Work habitually at maximum effort, taking muscles and joints to their fullest use – with much deep breathing and perspiration.	3 Be able to lead, follow, mirror and copy a partner's movements exactly.	3 Make short dances with clear beginnings, middles and ends.
4 Plan, compose and present short dances with an understanding of elements of 'Style' – variety, contrasts, and skilful movement.	4 Perform compositions created by self and others with good form, style and clear technical demands.	4 Express feelings, moods and ideas and create simple characters and stories in response to a range of stimuli, as in 'Good Samaritan'.
5 Accompany short sequences with vocal accompaniment to stimulate contrasting actions.	5 Express 'Winter' in movement, responding to seasonal words, percussion, and help from an observing partner.	5 Learn and perform a folk dance from outside the British Isles, e.g. a less vigorous, more relaxed and gesture-filled Caribbean dance.
6 Respond imaginatively to varied challenges and stimuli, showing increasing skill, versatility and an awareness of 'movement'.	6 Be whole-body conscious in expressing movement qualities, in a 'larger than life' way.	6 Work in groups to plan, practise and remember longer dances in response to varied stimuli. Such dances often include a teacher-directed start and finish, and a group-created middle, as in 'In The Mood' and 'Rock 'n' Roll'.
7 Create a seasonal autumn dance such as 'Autumn Trees', with a vocal accompaniment to varied movement qualities in trunk, branches and leaves.	7 Plan and perform own traditional-style dance, using four of the figures taught, in a 32-bar repeating dance.	7 Work whole-heartedly and with enthusiasm, increasingly stamping performances with own special style and personality.
8 Show ability to recognise, then pass on a movement to another, emphasising clearly its main features.	8 Learn, improve and remember a well-known, popular British Isles folk dance.	8 Give an impression of confidence and concentration, always trying to improve and achieve.
9 Make well-informed comments on another's work.	9 Be physically active for own sake; mindful of others for their sake; and proud of good footwork and good teamwork in folk dance.	9 Observe a performance, pick out good-quality features and make helpful, encouraging comments.
	10 Express moods and ideas and create simple characters in a story like 'City Life'.	
	11 Compare two performances and indicate differences in content and effectiveness.	

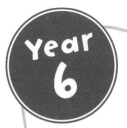

Year 6

Lesson Plan 1 • 30 minutes
September

Theme: *Rhythmic patterns.*

Warm-up Activities
5 minutes

1 Show me your best stepping in time with this medium-speed music. If I beat my drum loudly on count eight each time, can you introduce a change – style or size of step, body shape, firmness of whole body, or direction, for example? Best stepping, go! Best stepping, spacing well, 5, 6, 7 and change! Keep practising.

2 Well done. I saw changes to step size; stepping with high knees; stepping and closing sideways (as in folk dance chasse); sliding steps; stepping with feet apart; and very relaxed and very firm stepping.

3 Leaping is like high, wide running or stepping. Do four lively leaps, then four 'easy' actions on the spot. Go! Leap and leap and leap for 4; on the spot, 3, 4; leap high, leap long, for 3, for 4; easy action, 3, 4; leap and leap and leap for 4; keep going.

4 I liked your contrasting big/lively and small/easy movements.

Movement Skills Training
12 minutes

1 Still working in groups of eight counts, can you stay on the spot and show me a pattern of favourite actions or movements? May I suggest stepping, bouncing, skipping, clapping, gesturing or turning? Two or more actions, neatly linked and contrasting, will be excellent. Go! On the spot, on the spot, 5, 6, 7 and change; new action, contrast action, 5, 6, 7, again!

2 Well done. That looked really good and I enjoyed the many shapes as you put your whole body into it.

3 Now for favourite travelling actions. We have used steps and leaps of all sorts. You might want to add skipping, bouncing, running and galloping. Can you show me your varied travelling pattern, with eight counts to each one? Go! Travel, 2, 3, 4, 5, 6, 7, change; new travel, 3, 4, 5, 6, change again!

Dance — Patterns on a Stage
12 minutes

1 The middle third of the hall is going to be your stage for the final part of our lesson. It extends from side to side, from this line to that line and is quite big.

2 Start off the stage, walk to the edge of the stage and then do a two-part travelling action pattern to take you on to the stage. On the spot, you will then do your two-part pattern. After that, you will make your way off-stage to the other end with the same, or a different, two-part travelling action pattern.

3 While you are waiting off-stage, look for a good space before you come on-stage again to repeat your three patterns – the travelling on-stage; the on-the-spot; and the travelling from the stage.

4 I will stand at the side of your stage to watch your on-stage performance. Pretend I am a talent scout and do your very best.

5 Each half of the class will now watch the other half from the side of the stage. Spectators, you may quietly clap any impressive performance as the dancer leaves the stage, and be able to tell us what you particularly liked about him or her.

6 Spectators, look for neat movements using the whole body in larger than life activity; good, clear, proud body shapes; and varied use of directions and body tension, both firm and gentle.

Dance

Teaching notes and NC guidance
Development over 3 lessons

Pupils should be taught to:

a recognise the safety risks of wearing inappropriate jewellery, footwear and clothing
b respond readily to instructions
c be mindful of others
d adopt the best possible posture and use of the body
e be physically active.

This checklist of essential features should be established, if necessary, with a class at the start of a new school year. The highest possible standards of safety, progress and achievement will never be achieved if a class:

○ is badly dressed, wearing jewellery; long leg coverings that catch heels; large, noisy ungiving 'trainers'; or unbunched long hair that impedes vision;
○ behaves badly by incessantly talking; failing to listen and respond to instructions – particularly to 'Stop!';
○ contains anti-social elements who rush around at high speed, disturbing others, selfishly ignoring the need of others for a reasonable space to work in; and who do not work co-operatively in partner or group work;
○ slouch lazily through the lessons, standing, sitting or moving with sagging posture; never trying whole-heartedly to show a strong, firm, clear shape; never trying to look good;
○ continually works at less than maximum effort; never takes muscle and joint actions to their fullest use; and never gives the impression of breathing deeply and perspiring profusely.

Warm-up Activities

1–2 Stepping to the eight-beat phrasing of the music continues after the drum-inspired 'Change!' The teacher helps pupils' planning of 'changes' with reminders of those elements in Dance that provide variety, contrast and improved quality – style and size of steps; body shapes; direction of travel; and effort and body tension being used.

3–4 Running and jumping with a high, vigorous leap, alternating with gentler, on-the-spot actions is a teacher-directed, further example of a contrasting change of action.

Movement Skills Training

1–2 The teacher emphasises that you need two or three different actions within a sequence or a pattern of movements – the lesson's theme. Several on-the-spot (and ideally contrasting) actions make the first pattern to be planned and practised. Praise needs to be specific, rather than simply 'That was good' if the class are to learn from it and progress. 'I enjoyed the many shapes as you put your whole body into it.'

3 The reference to 'shapes' 'and 'whole body involvement' will provide good ideas to include in the patterns of travelling actions. By now, after five primary school years and much pupil experience of travelling actions, the teacher should be kept very busy, recognising, praising and demonstrating patterns of neat, quiet, controlled repeating sequences of travelling.

Patterns on a Stage Dance

The teacher will often have told the class that the hall is like a stage for them to perform and present on. Now, their stage is the middle third of the hall to approach; travel on to with a two-action pattern; perform on with two actions; and then travel away from with the same or a new pattern of travelling actions.

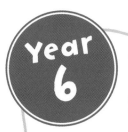

Lesson Plan 2 • 30 minutes
September/October

Theme: *Voice sound accompaniment.*

Warm-up Activities
5 minutes

1 No music today! Let's share the voice sound accompaniment in our warm-ups. Feet astride, slowly str-e-e-t-ch every part of your body. You say the next action and decide whether it will be v-e-r-y s-l-o-w or sudden. Go!

2 Once again, my slow str-e-e-t-ch. Now your turn. Go!

3 With me, st-e-e-p-p-ing plus st-re-e-t-ching, ultra-slow motion with a long stretch in arms, legs and body. Now your travel with a body action – slow motion, normal speed or fast forward. Go!

4 Let's combine the two pairs of actions with our voices making the accompaniment and the rhythm, on the spot, then moving.

Movement Skills Training
15 minutes

We accompanied ourselves, doing big movements on the spot and travelling, at normal speed, fast and slow. Remember when composing a dance to include the following:

a Jumping. Try on the spot; after a run; from one foot to both; from one to other; two to two; and with wide, long or twisted shapes.

b Turning. Do one on the spot, then one around an enclosed space. Turns are usually long, slow, graceful movements and different parts can lead you – elbow, back, side, shoulder, back of one hand.

c Rising and falling. From a low, still, crouched or lying start, you rise up to start or continue the dance. From upright, can you lower or fall to finish at floor level?

d Open and close. Contrast the opening action of sowing and scattering seeds with the closing action, pulling in a fisherman's nets, in a harvest or sea dance.

e Gesture. Show movements by body parts not supporting weight. A gesture can be expressive: goal!; despair with shoulders sagging; anger with a stamp; surprise with hands suddenly lifted.

f Stillness. Before start; often at the end; sometimes within the dance. Body shape varies, depending on the nature of the movement preceding or following. Be still! Travel... and be still!

Dance — Spa-a-ghe-e-tti Bo-o-ol-ogn-e-ese!
10 minutes

1 Use some of the activities we have just practised as you move to different parts of 'Spaghetti Bolognese', making some parts sl-oo-w and lo-o-o-ng, and some parts quick and maybe explosive. Have a practice, saying the words clearly.

2 Remember to use some of the activities we practised earlier. Can you include, at least, a travel, a jump and stillness?

3 Well done. Now add in a turn, rise and fall, or open and close.

4 Pretend you own an Italian restaurant and are trying to attract lots of customers. Make your dance very expressive and eye-catching as you dance and talk your way through it. Go!

5 Very well done. I particularly liked Theo's final gesture with one arm forwards, as if holding a tray for us to admire, almost saying 'I'm the best!'

6 Let's have half of the class looking at and listening to the other half to share all these brilliant ideas.

Dance

Teaching notes and NC guidance
Development over 3 lessons

Pupils should be taught to:

a respond readily to instructions. The warm-up and the middle part of the lesson contain much direct teaching, with the class being told about ten things to do in reasonably quick succession. An immediate, whole-hearted and thoughtful response is essential. The planning and performing of the dance climax also requires pupils to listen carefully to the precise details of the challenge, so they can be imaginative and creative during the pupil-centred section of the lesson.

b be physically active. It might be appropriate for the teacher to tell the class 'Year 6 is the very best age for Physical Education. You are strong and supple, and able to learn skills quicker and better than at any subsequent age. Once a skill is learned by your body it is remembered for a very long time. Please use this school year to work hard in all our lessons and learn as many enjoyable, healthy, sociable and worthwhile physical skills as possible.'

Pupils should be able to show that they can respond imaginatively to the various challenges. Year 6 pupils can be tremendously imaginative, and another reason for insisting on 'immediate responses to instructions', is the need to make time for demonstrations. Knowing that they will be asked to demonstrate inspires pupils to greater effort, and the demonstrations increase the repertoire of teacher and class.

Warm-up Activities

1–4 This double challenge needs pupils' instant attention and thoughtful participation. They have to plan both their whole-body, on-the-spot warm-up action, and the accompanying vocal sound. The teacher demonstrates the starting action and vocal sound. 'Me... you!' The teacher's second action, stepping and stretching slowly, possibly in ultra-slow motion, and the teacher's accompanying vocal sounds, continues the warm-up, and each class member now has to plan his or her own travelling action and vocal sounds. The a: b: c: d repeating pattern includes: teacher's actions and sounds on the spot; pupils' actions and sounds on the spot; teacher's travelling actions and vocal sounds; class travelling actions and vocal sounds.

Movement Skills Training

The teacher can ask the class 'If we pass, catch, shoot and dribble in basketball, what do you think we do in Dance? Tell me some of the things you remember from all your Dance lessons.' Each answer given is followed by a reminder of good practice in the action. Travelling; jumping; rising and falling; and gesture should all be easily recalled. 'Stillness' and 'Opening and closing' might not have been considered as 'content', and practice is needed to show good examples of their use. Opening and closing are excellent whole-body contrasts. Stillness before and after working, with the body shape showing what is about to happen or what has just happened, can provide an attractive, poised start and finish for a dance.

Spa-a-ghe-e-tti Bo-o-ol-ogn-e-ese! Dance

In the build up to their voice sounds-led dance, pupils are encouraged to include travelling, jumping and stillness from the seven actions already practised. Turning, and rising and falling, are added, and can accompany long, slow parts of the expanding words as a balance to sudden jumps and gestures.

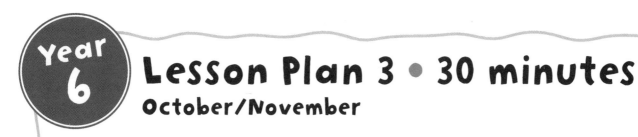

Lesson Plan 3 • 30 minutes
October/November

Theme: *Autumn.*

Warm-up Activities
5 minutes

1 Thomas, on top of the high box, is going to throw the leaves I brought in, as high as he can. Watch how they fly in many different ways – particularly with the windows open, to help their flight. Pretend they have just left their branches.

2 Can you try to show me some of the movement qualities seen during their flight? Off you go, flying, gliding, tilting, turning, hovering in unpredictable pathways and directions.

3 Your movements are free, light, sometimes being carried a long way, then held almost on the spot before soaring down and rising quickly.

4 You should all have a different shape like my leaves. Are you flat, crinkly, curled, long, wide, twisted or jagged? Show me.

5 One last flight, please. Think about your shape, light travelling actions, speed changes, and all the spaces you visit. Go!

Movement Skills Training
12 minutes

1 I enjoyed your wildly unpredictable leaf-like movements. Show me how you might express the movements of a branch on a tree. Can you start in a shape to represent your choice of branch – long, thin and 'bendy'; solid, heavy, unbending; or medium size with lots of lesser, intertwining, branches sprouting in all directions?

2 Show me the distances you think your kind of branch might move in space.

3 Are your movements fast, slow, strong, gentle, or a mixture that depend on the force of the wind and your size and weight?

4 Are some of you able to intertwine with one or both arms with a nearby branch?

Dance — Autumn Trees
13 minutes

1 Show me how you might express the restricted, strong movement of the tree trunk at the heart of our tree. Grip the floor firmly with your feet (roots) and move slowly and firmly.

2 Your speed will be far slower than the branches or leaves and will involve your whole body as it sways in all directions.

3 Practise again your branch-like movements, which depend on your size and shape. Feel the greater freedom and greater distances travelled after the very restricted trunk-like movements. Intertwine with a similar branch next to you, if you like.

4 Change to practising movements that express the very free, light, variable speeds of leaves in flight.

5 For our 'Autumn Trees' dance, there will be three groups: the trunk group at the centre; the branches group as an inner circle; and the outside leaves group, attached at first, then breaking free and flying away. Practise your actions and see if they can be fitted into a repeating pattern. Can you include a voice accompaniment as we did in the previous lesson? Creaking trunks, groaning branches, swooshing leaves?

6 Be ready to start, everyone. Build up from a soft, gentle wind, to medium strength, to a raging gale with increasing volume sound accompaniment. Good movement and good sound, please. Begin!

Dance

Teaching notes and NC guidance
Development over 3 lessons

Physical Education should involve pupils in: the continuous process of planning, performing and evaluating. The greatest emphasis should be placed on the actual performance. It is fair and sensible to put the class 'in the picture' regarding the aims of each new lesson, particularly if there is to be some assessment of their achievement. They should be told the nature of the hoped-for achievement.

'In National Curriculum Physical Education, the three most important headings are planning, performing and evaluating. In all your lessons I want to feel that you are planning, thinking ahead, and making your own good decisions about what actions to do, where to do them, and how to do them.

'We are lucky in Physical Education because it is easy to see the whole class performing from all parts of the room. I want to see you working hard to give a neat, quiet, well-controlled, poised performance – and able to remember and repeat it for me.

'"Evaluating" means that you watch others performing or think about your own work, and then make helpful comments about what you liked, about the important features and quality of the movements, and maybe suggest ways in which the performance can be improved.

'In our "Autumn Leaves" dance, you will be asked to plan and show me the three very different kinds of movement typical of the tree trunk, its branches and its leaves. I will look forward to seeing (and listening) to your stylish performances. Then, each of the three groups in turn will perform and be watched by the other two, who will reflect on what impressed them. The helpful comments and suggestions will then be used to improve our next practice.'

Warm-up Activities

1–4 Even better than using their imagination as a guide to performing in a certain way is the actual observation of the items themselves in action. Pupils will see and immediately copy the special, widely varied qualities of the leaves in flight. Practising the movements and assuming the shapes is easier, after observation, than reading or hearing about them. We remember what we see – the soaring, gliding, hovering, directions, speeds and shapes.

Movement Skills Training

1–4 The teacher challenges their imagination and creativity with 'Show me...'; 'Can you...?'; 'Are your movements fast, slow..., strong, gentle...?' The leaves, here, practising for the start of the dance, are still attached to a branch.

Autumn Leaves Dance

1–2 'Show me the strong movement of the tree trunk' produces slow, restricted, firm movements that contrast with the livelier, freer leaf movements already practised. Every part of the body needs to be used to represent the trunk. Some leaf movements were able to be expressed by the fingers and arms only. The trunk is a slow moving fixture with only slight movements.

3–4 Freer movements of branches, and livelier, lighter flying movements of leaves are revised.

5–6 The three groups of the dance climax include: the tree trunk centre; the branches inner circle; and the leaves perimeter. They build up from a gentle wind to a raging gale, accompanying themselves with an increasing volume of vocal sounds to match the increasingly large movements.

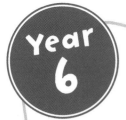

Lesson Plan 4 • 30 minutes
November

Theme: *Contrasts in body tension.*
Music: *Kitchen Sink.*

Warm-up Activities
5 minutes

1 This slow *Eastenders*-style music, with its eight-count phrasing, is perfect for slow travelling steps and big movements. Step slowly to the music. Slow, slow, 3, 4, 5, 6, keep on going.

2 Add a full body bend and stretch as you travel. You can stretch on the odd numbers, bend on the evens. Go! Stretch and bend for 3 and 4, stretch and bend for 7, repeat.

3 For variety, can you reach out, up or down for your stretches and bendings, always accompanied by your slow, rhythmic stepping?

Movement Skills Training
12 minutes

Phrase 1: Stretching out strongly and curling back gently.

1 Sit down near a partner, without touching, in a position from which you can move your whole body into a full, firm stretch.

2 Which part of your body will lead into your stretch? (An arm, leg or one of each, probably.) Ready? Stretch firmly, 3 and 4. Hold your whole-body stretch with no sagging parts.

3 Curl in gently and take four counts to arrive. Let the curl come right in towards your middle. Ready? Curl in, 3 and 4.

Phrase 2: Stretch strongly, curl back gently, but with a different part or parts stretching out into a different shape. The easy, gentle curl back ends in a kneeling position, all facing front. Stretch firmly, 3, 4; curl back gently, kneel to face the front.

Phrase 3: Right hand stretch up, left hand stretch up, curl back to starting position (four counts up, four counts down). Kneel tall, facing front and stretch strongly upwards, 1 and 2, with your right hand. Left hand follows, 3 and 4. Both arms gently curl down together, returning to position as at start of dance, four counts.

Phrases 4 and 5: Repeat phrases 1 and 2.

Phrase 6: Walk to meet your partner, ready for shared stretches. All travel for six counts, meet partner and go down into the very first position during counts seven and eight.

Phrases 7 and 8: Stretch out firmly and contact partner with a body part. Curl in gently. Stretch out strongly again, making contact again. Curl in and hold your final position still (illustrated).

Dance — Stretching and Curling
8 minutes

1 Sit near your partner. Stretch up and curl down, eight counts.

2 Stretch up and curl down, with a different body part stretching up.

3 Kneel, all facing the front, right hand stretch up, left hand stretch up, both hands curl back down.

4 Stretch up and bend down; stretch up and bend down.

5 Walk to meet your partner. From dance start position, stretch with body contact with your partner twice. Finish, curled still.

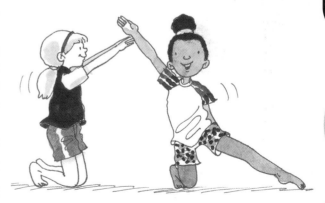

Dance

Teaching notes and NC guidance
Development over 3 lessons

Pupils should be taught to:

a respond to music;

b respond to a range of stimuli through Dance. Music is one of the many varied stimuli used to make lessons interesting. In Year 6 these include: actions, patterns, voice sounds, nature, percussion, country-dance steps and figures, follow the leader, a Bible story and work actions. The slow *Eastenders*-style music inspires slow whole-body movements that contrast with the much quicker music of other lessons;

c compose and control their movements by varying shape, size, level and tension. With the short phrasing of the music, it is easy to repeat, practise and refine the firm, strong, whole-body stretches with different parts to different levels, and to contrast them with the more gentle curling back in to oneself.

Pupils should be able to show that they can repeat sequences with increasing control and accuracy. This is a short dance with a few, simple movements. The movements are performed slowly, allowing lots of time to do each one carefully and thoughtfully. Demonstrations, with couples observing other couples, lead to a sharing of good ideas. The teacher's accompanying rhythm serves both as a reminder of what is happening, and an encouragement to achieve greater quality. 'Stretch out strongly, whole body firm; curl back gently, easily for four.'

Warm-up Activities

1–3 This practice gives a feel for the slow rhythm which will be an ever-present feature of the lesson. Pupils are more used to moving at a medium speed or to a lively rhythm. Unusually, the very slow travelling speed lets them include bendings and stretchings within the travelling.

Movement Skills Training

Phrase 1–2: (All seated beside a partner, able to do a firm whole-body stretch up, and able to see the teacher.) The dance is short enough, and danced slowly enough, to let the teacher, starting off kneeling at the front, demonstrate and lead the class through the whole dance. His or her accompanying commentary emphasises the contrasting movements which are the main feature of the dance: 'Stretch strongly, 3, 4; curl in gently, 3, 4; new strong stretch, 3, 4; curl back softly, 3, 4.'

Phrase 3: (All kneeling tall, facing the teacher.) 'Right hand, strongly stretch; left hand, strongly stretch; both arms softly curl, 3, 4.'

Phrases 4 and 5: Repeat phrases 1 and 2.

Phrase 6: (Rise to standing for short walkabout, circling for six counts before returning to starting, seated position beside partner on counts 7 and 8.) 'Slowly walk for 3, 4, 5, 6, sit beside your partner.'

Phrases 7 and 8: 'Stretch firmly to contact partner; softly in; stretch again to contact, gently in.'

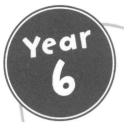

Year 6

Lesson Plan 5 • 30 minutes
December

CD TRACK 6

Theme: *Christmas and sharing.*

Warm-up Activities
5 minutes

1   Stand facing a partner, about two metres apart. One starts as leader, the other watches and mirrors the actions and movements shown. The music is medium/slow to help you keep together. Start off, leader, with an action on the spot, using your legs. Go!

2   Can you make your action travel, for example to one side, then back; or to leader's rear, then forwards? Mirroring partner goes the opposite way, of course.

3   Once again, perform on the spot, then travel, then on the spot, then travel, making a repeating pattern.

4   Do it all again with the following partner adding a simple, accompanying body movement for the original leader to copy. It can be a simple clapping on the spot and a gesturing of arms on the move – or something more adventurous if you like.

5   We might call this 'A double follow the leader' or 'Two mirrors on a moving wall'. Well done. Keep practising.

Movement Skills Training
15 minutes

1   Start in a big circle where you can all see me. Listen to the rhythmic, medium/slow tempo of the music and all say with me 'Watch it, pass it on', keeping with the beat of the music.

2   Watch my simple action as you say 'Watch it' and then copy it as you say 'Pass it on.'

3   Watch it again on the 'Watch it', but on the 'Pass it on' turn to the person on your right and present the action in their direction. This gives practice in the passing on, even if that person is busy doing the same thing to his or her right.

4   Watch me carefully as I do a four-part routine, with each action being shown once only. 'Watch it (for example, a handclap), pass it on, watch it (for example, a small step forwards and back with one foot), pass it on, watch it (for example, knees bend and stretch), pass it on, watch it (for example jump to wide position, arms stretched), Pass it on.' Very well done. Most of you kept with me and passed it on.

5   Will anyone volunteer to think of four actions to lead the class through, please? Thank you, Grace. We are all ready for our next 'Watch it, pass it on.' Begin when you are ready, please.

6   Thank you, Grace, and well done. Can we have a boy volunteer now, please? Thank you, Liam. Start when ready, please.

Dance – Pass the Movement Parcel
10 minutes

1   Make circles of five. Your leader will do a four-action repeating sequence, calling out 'Watch it, pass it on.' Begin.

2   That was easy. Now, with a new leader, try the more difficult passing on, only to the next person. Number two watches the leader and passes it on to number three, who watches it and passes it on to number four, who passes it on to number five. After two has passed it on, he or she looks back at the leader to see the new action, then passes it on to number three, who watches it and passes it on to number four, and so on. Eventually the 'passed on' actions come back to the leader, who continues to pass them on.

3   Let's have a look at each 'Passing on' circle in turn.

Dance

Teaching notes and NC guidance
Development over 3 lessons

Pupils should be taught to:

a respond readily to instructions. This lesson, with its three stages of development – 'mirroring another'; 'watching another and passing it on'; and a group 'watching and passing it on' – is quite difficult and requires concentration and attention, by everyone, for an enjoyable and successful outcome.

b be mindful of others. 'Others' include a partner to whom you are showing good quality movements of which your partner is capable; the partner whose actions you are mirroring to the best of your ability for joint success; the teacher in the middle of the lesson on whom you are concentrating totally; and your team-mates in the dance climax for whom you are trying the hardest, before the inevitable demonstration by your group.

c respond to a range of stimuli through Dance. Lesson by lesson, increasingly varied stimuli make Dance lessons more interesting, exciting and enjoyable. Eventually, the varied challenges make the dancers more skilful and versatile. The topical, Christmas 'Pass the Movement Parcel!' dance is completely different from anything they have done before.

Pupils should be able to show that they can practise, improve and refine performance. A suggested approach to practising and improving performance is to have a three-stage development plan:

1 clarify the actions, the body parts concerned and the clear shapes
2 add interest by varying directions, levels and good use of the space all around
3 clarify the amount of effort or speed that is right.

Warm-up Activities

1–5 This follow-the-leader is a facing 'mirror the leader' who does a simple action on the spot, using legs, followed by a simple travel action. The actions need to be simple because the follower has to add another movement to each, for the original leader to copy into their 'Double follow the leader' four-part repeating pattern of mirrorings.

Movement Skills Training

1–6 The whole class need to say 'Watch it, pass it on' several times until they can keep to the slow/medium beat of the accompanying music. They progress to watching the teacher's simple action on 'Watch it' and copying the action on 'Pass it on.' The next stage is to pretend that they are passing it on to the one on their right as they look at that person on the 'Pass it on.' A four-part routine, watching and pretending to pass on the teacher's four actions to the one on their right, needs their full attention. The biggest problem is the responding at the same time as the teacher (as in the earlier mirroring) instead of watching and then responding. Volunteers are challenged to plan a routine of four repeating actions for the whole class to watch and then follow.

Pass the Movement Parcel Dance

In circles of five with a leader, the leader's actions, one at a time, are passed on anti-clockwise to number two, who passes it on to number three and so on around the circle. Each passes on an action, then looks again at the passer for the next action.

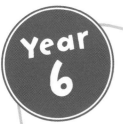

Lesson Plan 6 • 30 minutes
January

Theme: *Winter.*

CD TRACK 5

Warm-up Activities
5 minutes

1   With a partner, do 'Follow the leader' where the leader shows lively, travelling actions that use every joint to warm you up. Keep in time with the medium-speed music. Go!

2   Stop! The other partner will now lead in whole body, lively actions on the spot. Once again, try to use every joint and muscle in your body. Try to mirror your leader exactly. Begin!

3   In your two-part winter warm-up, travel to a good space, then face each other for your on-the-spot actions. Keep with the phrasing of the music as you do your repeating patterns. Go!

Movement Skills Training
15 minutes

1   Your deeper breathing and perspiring faces tell me that you warmed up successfully. Well done. One of your couple will now collect a piece of percussion while the other collects one of my three different sets of cards with their three winter words.
    Set 1: Birds in winter wind FLUTTER SOAR SWIRL
    Set 2: Snow DRIFT FREEZE MELT
    Set 3: People STAMP SLIP SHIVER

2   Put your card down on the floor. Study the words and plan how your movements will clearly represent the words.

3   Number one dancer, practise your three actions clearly for your partner to watch. Start when ready, without any percussion.

4   Dancer, your partner will give you one helpful comment to improve your performance. Were the actions correct? Did they express clearly the main movement qualities of the actions? Were the shapes clear? Was the timing too hurried or too slow?

5   Same dancer again, please, accompanied by partner on percussion. Percussionist, quietly accompany your partner, starting and stopping each time to make the three actions separate.

6   Well done. The improvements were obvious. Now change places.

7   New dancers, stand ready, please. No accompaniment yet as partner watches to see what might be improved. Begin when ready.

8   Dancers, your partner will tell you one thing that might be improved. Can the main movement feature be expressed better? Can the whole body be more involved? What about an exciting contrast in effort or speed?

9   Same dancers with percussion this time. Each action is started and stopped by the percussion. Start when ready, please.

10 Well done, dancers and partners whose advice produced an obvious improvement.

Dance – Winter Words with Percussion
10 minutes

1   I have placed your couple next to a couple with a different set of winter words. Hide your card so they can't read the words.

2   Each couple in turn will perform twice, working as dancer and percussionist to see if the other couple recognise your words.

3   Do it all again. Observers, please watch and then tell the other couple what you particularly liked in their demonstrations.

Dance

Teaching notes and NC guidance
Development over 3 lessons

Pupils should be taught to:

a adopt the best possible posture and use of the body. We want the dancers to be conscious of their whole body in expressing the different qualities of their three action words. Before they start, they should be asked 'Show me by your starting posture what your first action is.' Arms, shoulders, head and spine, as well as legs, all need to be used to express the lightweight, hovering, 'flutter'; the gentle, travelling 'drift'; or the firm, heavy 'stamp'.

b respond readily to instructions. The short sequences will only be improved by listening carefully and responding to the helpful, general teaching points and individual coaching by the teacher, and by trying to respond to the one main suggestion for improvement made by the partner.

c respond to a range of stimuli, through Dance. The three-fold stimuli include seasonal action words, percussion, and an observing partner/coach, in addition to the ever-present stimulus of an enthusiastic, appreciative teacher.

Pupils should be able to show that they can make simple judgements about another's performance to improve the accuracy, quality and variety of the performance. The observing percussion partner can be asked 'Please put up your hand if you think your dancer improved as a result of your advice. You will then be asked to identify the improvement.'

Warm-up Activities

1 This partners' winter warm-up requires big, lively, travelling whole-body actions with the leader doing his or her best to 'use every joint to warm you up.' Arms and legs will be lifting, swinging, bending, stretching to the full range of their possible movement.

2 Partners are challenged to mirror each other on the spot with the new leader encouraged to show whole-hearted, whole-body actions for partner to follow, with particular emphasis on many joints, from ankles up to upstretched arms, stretching and bending fully and powerfully.

3 The two parts of the sequence each have two parts – travel; travel; on the spot; on the spot, with each leader leading twice.

Movement Skills Training

This lesson's development is easy, straightforward and popular because of the use of percussion and the excellent partner co-operative activity. The pattern is as follows:

1 Partners put card on floor, study the words and plan how they will represent them.

2 Dancer practises to teacher's timing. 'First action... go! Second action... go! Third action... go!' Dancer is watched by partner who will be providing some helpful coaching.

3 Dancer sits beside observing partner to be told something encouraging and something that will be an improvement.

4 Dancer repeats the three actions, with the percussion accompaniment setting the times for each of the words.

5 Whole process is repeated with other partner as dancer and coach/percussionist.

Percussion players are asked to pause in between playing for each action to make partner listen, concentrate, prepare, then respond to the next sound.

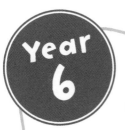

Lesson Plan 7 • 30 minutes
February

Theme: *Creative, traditional folk-dance.*

Warm-up Activities
5 minutes

1 Take eight steps of the music to travel from space to space. Use any steps, including some you make up. Arrive in your new space on eight and dance on the spot for eight, using steps we have learned or your own creation. Travelling, and on the spot, in counts of eight, go!

2 Stop! Join with a partner, dance together to your next space, then do eight steps on the spot. One leads with the follower remembering the steps. Follower leads on the spot with partner remembering.

3 Each of you decided a part of the dance, watched by the other. Can you now keep going, copying actions as you travel, and then as you stay – always using eight counts of the music for each?

New Figures for Groups of Four
15 minutes

Make a square of four dancers anywhere in the room. This is not a set with first and second couples. It is simply a group of four who will not travel outside their own floor space area as you try some new ideas for folk dance figures, taking eight counts.

a 1 dances to 2's position with two travelling steps.
2 dances to 4's position.
4 dances to 3's position.
3 dances to 1's position.
Repeat in the other direction for 8 more counts, 1 starting.

b 1 and 4 dance to change places for 2 counts.
2 and 3 dance to change places.
1 and 4 return to own places.
2 and 3 return to own places.

c 1 and 4 make an arch with hands joined for 2 and 3 to dance under to change places for 4 counts.
Arch remains for 2 and 3 to dance back to places for 4 counts.
Repeat with 2 and 3 making an arch for 1 and 4.

d 3 and 2 join hands for a tiny circle left and right.
1 and 4 dance in a bigger circle, 4 counts to the right and 4 back to left to own places.

e 1 leads 2 across, outside the line of 3 and 4 and back around square to own side and starting places for 8 counts.
Repeat with 3 leading 4 across and around the square for 8 counts.

f Can you think of any other interesting figure that does not take you away from your own group floor space?

Groups of Four Plan and Practise Own 32-bar Dance
10 minutes

Four figures will be linked together and it is good to have everyone dancing for the last 8 counts. This might be the one you create as your climax. For example, all step forwards, joining and raising hands to a peak, then stepping out backwards. Good ideas will be demonstrated, shared, praised and sometimes copied.

Dance

Teaching notes and NC guidance
Development over 3 lessons

Pupils should be involved in the continuous process of planning, performing and evaluating, and the greatest emphasis should be on the actual performances. Planning and creativity can both be indulged in a folk dance setting. The class repertoire will ideally include 'modern' folk dances in addition to those from 'different times and places'.

Pupils should be taught to:

a respond to music. The eight-bar phrasing in the warm-up; the eight-count figures of the middle of the lesson; and the four by eight-bar extent of the created dance, all make the class aware of the beat to be followed. Teacher chanting helps to keep the dancers in time with the music, and is a reminder of what is happening. 'Your first figure, 3, 4, 5, 6, ready to change; second figure, 3, 4, 5, 6, third figure, now...'.

b perform a number of dances, including some traditional dances of the British Isles. The music here is traditional, as is the travelling step and the slipping step sideways in the circle. The figures are traditional, as pupils change places, make arches to go under, circle to the left and right, or cast off to their own side. The four-figure repeating pattern of the dance is traditional. It is hoped that the excellent posture, the dancing in time with the music, and the sociable togetherness and excellent teamwork typical of good folk dance, are also in evidence.

Pupils should be able to show that they can:

a work safely, sensibly, co-operatively and unselfishly as members of a team. Such an attainment will be expressed in a poised team performance that flows smoothly from start to finish.

b repeat sequences with increasing control and accuracy. The music provides the rhythm and practice will enable the group to remember and repeat their four actions.

Warm-up Activities

1 An easy, instant start to folk dance music, travelling for 8 and dancing on the spot for 8.

2 Pairs travel together with one leading, one following. Follower leads partner on the spot.

3 This a: b; a: b; a: b; two-part, repeating pattern might be called a 'Dual follow my leader.'

New Figures for Groups of Four

a In the first figure, taking two counts, each pupil dances clockwise around to the next dancer's position. The whole circuit is repeated anti-clockwise, once again taking 8 counts.

b Dancers change places diagonally and then change places diagonally back to own places.

c A diagonally opposite pair make an arch for the other pair to go under to change places. This same pair go under again, back to own places. That travelling pair now make an arch for the other pair to go under, changing places, and then repeat, returning to own places.

d One diagonal pair, holding hands with bent arms, circle to left and to right. The other pair, at the same time, make a wide circle with long arms and circle to right and to left.

e Dancing pair, hands joined, circle around outside 3 and then 4, and return to own side of square. Other pair repeat the circling around and back to own places travelling.

Groups of Four Plan and Practise Own 32-Bar Dance

Ideally, each dancer will suggest one of the four figures needed for this 32 bar dance. A dance enthusiast might suggest a final, completely new figure, with all taking part, non-stop.

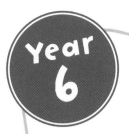

Lesson Plan 8 • 30 minutes
February/March

CD TRACKS 8 + 20

Theme: *Traditional folk dance.*

Warm-up Activities
5 minutes

1 Practise skip change of step with a partner who can be beside you, leading, following, or going away from and coming back to you. Let each action have eight counts of the music as a guide.

2 Show me neat foot movements as you hop at the start, then into your travel, 2, 3; lift, travel, 2, 3; lift, step, close up, step.

3 Can you decide which three or four ways you are going to relate to each other? Try to add interesting variety – together; apart; parting and meeting; one still, one going around.

Teach Figures of New Dance – Dashing White Sergeant
15 minutes

This is one of the most popular of all Scottish country dances, practised in sixes with three dancers facing three dancers. A boy between two girls faces a girl between two boys. Groups of sixes start in a circle formation around the room.

1 All six dancers join hands in a circle and dance eight slip steps to the left and eight back to the right.

2 Centre dancer, turn to right-hand partner. Set to each other and turn with both hands with four setting steps. Centre dancer, now do this with left-hand partner and finish facing to your right.

3 Dance a reel of three (figure of 8), centre dancer starting the reel by giving right shoulder to right hand partner. Eight skip changes of step to finish facing three dancers opposite.

4 All advance and retire, then pass on to meet the three dancers coming towards you, passing right shoulders with the person opposite.

Dance – Dashing White Sergeant
10 minutes

Music: *Dashing White Sergeant* or any lively 32-bar tune

Formation: A circle around the room in threes, one line of three facing clockwise and the other line of three facing anti-clockwise.

Bars 1–8 Circle left and right, eight slipping steps each way.

Bars 9–16 Centre dancer sets to and turns each of their partners.

Bars 17–24 Reel of three, to finish facing opposite trio.

Bars 25–32 Advance and retire and pass on to meet next three dancers and repeat the dance.

Dance

Teaching notes and NC guidance
Development over 3 lessons

Pupils should be taught to:

a be physically active, engaging in activities that develop the heart and the lungs. As well as being the most popular of all Scottish country dances, this is one of the most physical. The mixture of travelling, setting and slipping steps, all done at a lively speed, make it one of the most physically demanding. It is guaranteed to inspire deep breathing, lots of perspiration and much enjoyment.

b be mindful of others. The team element is high, with all six dancers needing to work and think hard to be in the right place at the right time, and to help one another by careful 'handling' as they place one another in the right positions.

c perform a number of dances from different times and places, including some traditional dances of the British Isles. This is a dance that expresses all that is good about lively folk dance. It is fun, friendly, physical; it depends on good team-work; performed well, it has beautiful flowing, attractive movement; and it has a long 'shelf life', able to be repeated and repeated.

Pupils should be able to show that they can repeat sequences with increasing control and accuracy. The music provides the guiding, lively rhythm. Good team-work, with all pupils thinking ahead, ensures the smooth repetition of the four-part pattern of the dance; and good teaching of one main point for each practice ensures an increase in quality.

Warm-up Activities

1–3 The basic travelling step, also known as 'skip change of step', needs to be constantly practised to ensure the 'Lift, travel, 2, 3; hop, 1, 2, 3; one foot forward, the other foot; hop, left, 2, 3; hop, right, 2, 3; change (leading) feet; change feet' pattern.

Teach Figures Of New Dance

1 Hands in the circle are joined at shoulder-height with hands above elbow-height. Because the slip steps to the left are fast, we slow down on six, and bring feet together on seven and eight, ready for the change of direction, under control, back to the right, for eight counts.

2 'Set to your right; turn for two; set to your left, turn for two.' The pairs of dancers help each other around in the complete turns on the 'turn for two' each time.

3 The reel of three, describing a figure of eight on the floor, needs to be practised at a slow walking pace first. It helps if the teacher joins in as the centre dancer, controlling the route to be followed around the figure, as a demonstration.

4 The two lines of three in each team can join hands as they advance and retire, then drop hands as they progress forwards to pass the trio with whom they have been dancing in the circle. If they 'pass right shoulders with the one opposite you' as they move on to join another trio, there will be no bumping of line into line.

Dashing White Sergeant Dance

The dance will be accompanied by the teacher's continuous chanting during the early practising: 'Circle left, 2, 3, 4, 5, 6, feet together; circle right, 2, 3, 4, 5, 6, ready to set; set to right for 2, turn for 2, set to left for 2, turn for 2; reel around, 3, 4, 5, 6, 7, join hands in lines; advance for 2, retire for 2, move past to meet the next group.'

Lesson Plan 9 • 30 minutes
March

Theme: *Creating a story with simple characters.*

Warm-up Activities
5 minutes

1 Listen to this anxious 'rushing around' music, then show me how you might respond to its urgent, somewhat jerky rhythm.

2 Well done. Lots of hither and thither, anxious looking, hurrying.

3 Can your anxiety include some watch watching to show that you might be late for something as you rush to your meeting place?

4 Be brilliant and produce a repeating pattern of anxious travelling to your destination. This is helped by pretending you are near home with streets, corners and crossings you know.

Movement Skills Training
15 minutes

1 Our movements represent a group of office workers. At the start our anxious travelling takes us to our bus stop, and we are a little late. All stand ready, at home, in an anxious shape.

2 We have decided the places you are travelling to, for your bus stop queues. Fifteen seconds of worried walking... go!

3 Stand in line at your bus stop. Lean forwards, looking right for the bus and looking at your watch. (Class in lines of four at the several bus stops, spaced around the room.)

Pattern: Look for the bus; look at your watch; stamp your feet, temper, temper! (Thrice.)

4 All step straight on to the bus, shoulder to shoulder, squashed, strap hanging with right hand, holding paper with left hand.

Pattern: Hang on your strap, hang on your strap; read your paper, read your paper; all stumble to the right. (One at the right-hand end stands firm.) Hang on your strap, hang on your strap; read the paper, read the paper; all stumble to the left. (Person at the left-hand end stands firm.) Three times, to right, to left, to right.

5 Off the bus and it is a short walk to the office where you all are half sitting at your desk, all in regimental lines, facing towards the same end.

Pattern: Pick up your phone; pick up your pen; listen to message; write it down, write it down. Phone down; pen down; type it up, type it up. File it high, file it high (into high drawer). Repeat.

6 Going home. Heavy feet. Tired city workers after a long day.

Dance — City Life
10 minutes

Five-part dance:

Time	
0 secs	To bus stop.
15 secs	In bus queue.
32 secs	On to bus.
50 secs	To office desk.
1min 18 secs	Home.
1min 30 secs	Dance ends.

Dance

Teaching notes and NC guidance
Development over 3 lessons

Pupils should be taught to:

a try hard to consolidate performances. Because the whole dance lasts only one and a half minutes, there are ample opportunities for improving, remembering, and being able to repeat the dance. It is recommended that during each practice or part of the dance, one teaching point only is emphasised. Right at the start the 'What?', or actions, should be clarified, with the body parts concerned and the shapes receiving a special focus. 'Where?', the next focus, considers the locations, possible changes of level or direction and ways to use one's own surrounding air space. 'How?', and interesting use of speed and effort, make a big contribution to the quality and variety of the performance.

b express feelings, moods and ideas.

c create simple characters and stories. The expression of the moods and feelings of the participants and their story are both done through movement. Imagery is used throughout to provide interest, understanding of what the dance is all about, and to conjure up easily visualised pictures. We move 'Like early morning commuters, with their anxious, rushing steps.' Our whole body moves 'Like an angry, stamping, bus queue person.' Imagery is used to help us visualise ourselves clearly in a real situation, and is better than the vague 'We are going to explore feelings. Can you show me "Anger"?' Imagery deserves to be included within the 'range of stimuli' that we are required to use in our teaching.

Warm-up Activities

1–4 The use of imagery and imagination helps to make pupils' expressions more 'real'. 'Pretend you are going to be late for work! Maybe your bus has gone. Check your watches.'

Movement Skills Training

1 The anxious Monday morning commuters look and act as if they might be too late for their usual bus. 'We hate Mondays!' might, also, be inferred through their desperate looks.

2–3 Lines of four, at their previously arranged bus-stop places, in unison look to their right, then re-check their watches, then, still together, stamp their feet angrily.

4 All hold newspaper in right hand, strap of bus in the left hand, and stumble, carefully, to the timing set by the teacher, thrice. End strap-hanger on side to which they are doing the little stumble, stands firmly to restrain the three stumblers.

5 'Off the bus and into your huge, open, office workplace, crouching as if sitting at your table, all facing me. Ready.' When they know the pattern for the office place, the teacher can shorten the explanation to 'Phone. Pen. Write order down. Phone down. Pen down. Type it up, type it up. File it high. File it high. (Repeat.)

6 Home time. Weary after their boring, repetitive day at their office tables. Expressing tiredness and complete lack of bounce in their steps.

City Life Dance

The progression is from a complete rehearsal of the dance with the teacher's non-stop reminder of all the actions to one where the teacher simply says 'Stand, ready to start with the music. If necessary, I will give you a short reminder of each part. Begin! Walk from home. At the bus stop. On the bus. Read and stumble; again. Off the bus into office. Phone and write. Phone and write. Go home.'

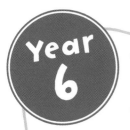

Lesson Plan 10 • 30 minutes
April

Theme: *Expressing feelings and creating a story.*

Warm-up Activities
5 minutes

1 Practise a punch, without any contact of course, and the reaction to it by your partner. Each of you take turns, reacting and staggering backwards.

2 Keep a safe distance apart and show me examples of punches to different parts of the body and the different reactions to them.

3 A punch towards the head has a violent, upper body, staggering reaction backwards. Be very careful. Try it – keeping well apart.

4 Good, punchers and reactors. Now, well apart, try a long distance kick towards your partner's abdomen. This should produce a crumpling, folding, extremely painful reaction.

5 Attacker, grab your partner by the shoulders or arms. Try a quick twist and a careful lowering of your partner, safely to the floor.

6 Well done, all couples. That was very sensibly practised and I saw many realistic actions.

Movement Skills Training
10 minutes

1 Join with another couple now and decide who is to be the victim, the puncher, the kicker, and the grabber and twister.

2 Victim, work in the field at your own choice of action – raking, digging or sowing. Attackers, spread out to surround the victim, ready for the attack.

3 Puncher, you come in from the front of the victim and your punch repels the victim backwards, turning him or her towards the kicker. The kick to the lower tummy crumples him or her. The third attacker reaches down and in, gripping on shoulders or arms, to twist and lower the victim all the way to the ground.

4 Please practise with great care, keeping a very safe distance apart on the punch and kick, and remembering to twist and lower the victim all the way to the floor. No judo throws!

5 May I see each group in turn to check on your safe actions and reactions.

Dance – The Good Samaritan
15 minutes

1 With your body movements, aim to express the feelings and emotions of the four groups.

2 Starting positions, please, with the victim working in the field.

3 Perform the fight sequence as we practised. Thieves, get into your attacking positions, surrounding the victim. Advance slowly and menacingly to punch, then kick, then grab and lower.

4 Victim lies wounded by the roadside. Thieves, walk away, moving towards the next victim, to represent another group on the busy road. You approach and look away as you come near this next victim. You 'pass by on the other side' pretending 'it's none of our business.'

5 Trios, move towards the next victim. This group expresses some concern. One bends to touch the victim, but all then 'pass by on the other side' again.

6 Trios, progress on to the next victim and your attitude shows a change for the better as you all try to help, in a disorganised way. One of you becomes leader and good Samaritan and organises the other two to lift the wounded victim very gently and slowly.

7 Victim, you are now strongly supported by the three encircling you, pushing you towards each other as their hands encourage life, movement and recovery.

8 In harmony, you all walk along together as friends, expressing compassion and caring.

9 Well done, everyone. You provided an interesting variety of expressions – the terrified victim; the cruel trio with their violence; the unconcerned; the semi-concerned, half-hearted, dithering third group; and the caring last group, led by the good Samaritan.

Dance

Teaching notes and NC guidance
Development over 3 lessons

'A certain man went down from Jerusalem to Jericho, and fell among thieves. They wounded him and departed, leaving him half dead. A priest saw him but passed by on the other side. A Levite came and looked at him and passed by on the other side. But a certain Samaritan saw him, had compassion and bound up his wounds. He set him on his own breast and took care of him.'

Pupils should be taught to:

a express feelings, moods and ideas.
b create simple ideas and stories. Feelings of aggression, menace, cruelty, pain, fear, disinterest, compassion and caring, as well as the story idea, are all expressed through whole-body movements that we associate with those feelings and that story.

Pupils should be able to show that they can work safely, sensibly, co-operatively and unselfishly as members of a team. By waiting nearly four years before including a dance expressing extreme aggression, it is hoped that the top year class will respond in a completely safe and sensible way to the instruction 'Never touch anyone!'

Warm-up Activities

1–6 Examples of an action and the reaction to it are practised at a safe one metre apart. The aggressive actions are easy and straightforward. The reactions by the victim are far more difficult to imagine and to practise, because most of the class will not have experienced and responded to such aggression. A whole-body tensing up to withstand the punch, the kick, or the grab is asked for. Legs need to feel strong, with feet apart to maintain balance.

Movement Skills Training

1 Groups of four are chosen to include one victim and three aggressors, each of whom is to use a different form of aggression.

2 The victim is busy, working in his or her field while the aggressors furtively spread out to surround the victim.

3–5 Careful choreography is needed, action by action, as the actions of the assailants and the reactions of the victim, are practised and improved, almost in slow motion. In the twist and lower of the third aggressor, a careful body contact, hands taking shoulders, is used for a gentle, slow movement.

The Good Samaritan Dance

1–3 A repetition of the work practised so far with the groups of four around the room.

4 Wounded victim lies by the roadside. The three thieving aggressors move away towards the next group in the hall to become a different group of travellers on the busy road. They approach and look at the next victim lying there and walk on without stopping to help.

5 As trios move on to where the next victim is lying, some concern is expressed, with one traveller bending to touch the victim, but they all pass by again.

6 In the next move, group by group, around the series of victims lying by the roadside, the approaching trio, disorganised at first, all show interest in trying to help the victim. The emerging Good Samaritan leader organises the two accompanying partners as they all slowly and gently lift the victim on to his or her feet.

7–9 Supporting hands encircle the victim, anxiously spreading recovery, affection and caring through warm, concerned hands. This expression of friendliness, concern and caring is further expressed as they all walk along together.

Year 6

Lesson Plan 11 • 30 minutes
May

CD TRACK 21

Theme: *Traditional folk dance.*

Warm-up Activities
5 minutes

Music: Lively Caribbean-style carnival or steel band music

1   The music is quite slow and your main body movement to start with is a lifting and lowering of each foot, keeping a flat 'lift and place' action going. 'One... and two; lift... and place.' The slowness of this action is made possible by a generous knee lift. 'Lift, then step; lift, then place; one... and two.'

2   Steps are done almost on the spot with little transfer forwards of weight. All practise this one step forwards per bar of music into a circle for eight; then backwards out for eight.

3   Repeat to centre with loose, free swings of the upper body and shoulders, with gestures to contrast with the simple little movements of the feet. Eight in to centre and eight back out again.

4   With feet still for four counts, bounce your knees, but with a generous lifting, lowering, and swinging of arms and shoulders. Travel forwards for four; do four on the spot; four backwards; and four on the spot.

Movement Skills Training
15 minutes

1   Do two steps to each bar of music. Step forwards on to flat right foot and put your weight on it. Bring the ball of your left foot up beside your right foot, but keep weight on right foot. Step forwards on to flat left foot and put your weight on it. Bring the ball of your right foot up beside your left, but keep weight on left foot. Step forwards on to right foot. Step, close; and step, close; and step, close, all into circle for eight and backwards out for eight.

2   Try one slow, followed by two quick. Step left... right, left; right... left, right; 1... 2, 3; 1... 2, 3; slow... quick, quick with one long and two short steps.

3   Show a partner your one or two patterns as you 'Follow the leader'. Let the upper body and arms work loosely and with big gestures since the feet are doing such simple movements.

4   You can be still for your start, simply letting upper body, arms and shoulders work loosely with little knee bounces, keeping the rhythm. Bounce... and bounce; loose arms and shoulders; bounce and bounce; now travel... and travel; one... and two.

Dance — Caribbean Maze
10 minutes

1   All follow me, keeping our big circle shape. It's important to keep following the person in front of you, as I lead you into a smaller and smaller circle, and then lead you out again. Go! (Teacher leads them around in the big starting circle, using the Caribbean steps already practised. The teacher goes inside those ahead of him or her to start a series of smaller circles. When the teacher runs out of space at the centre of the many concentric circles, he or she turns to go in the opposite direction, unwinding the many circles and re-creating the original circle. Clockwise into the maze is followed by anti-clockwise out from the maze.)

2   Well done. We got there. Now, in smaller circles of about eight dancers, let me see you making and unravelling your mazes.

Dance

Teaching notes and NC guidance
Development over 3 lessons

Pupils should be taught to:

a be physically active.

b adopt the best possible posture and use of the body. In actions with little travelling and a great deal of movement within the body, we focus as much on what the whole body is doing as on what the legs are doing. Upper body, shoulders and arms, swinging, lifting and turning, give the dance a lively physicality that compensates for the quiet leg actions.

c respond to music.

d perform a number of dances from different times and places. In the same way that the 'Dashing White Sergeant' music and dance give an excellent insight into the typical folk dance music and dance of Scotland, this music and dance express the less vigorous, more gesture-filled style of the Caribbean. The cold Scottish winters require a lively, vigorous dance, performed indoors. The warmer West Indies favour an outdoor, relaxed, carnival style.

Pupils should be able to show that they can repeat a series of movements performed previously. A repetitive pattern and rhythm are the main aids to practising, remembering, and being able to repeat sequences of movement. The smaller circles of the final part of the lesson will need to discuss, plan and agree the number of parts to their pattern, and decide how often to repeat each one.

Warm-up Activities

1–4 Unlike the usual travelling steps, with the body weight feeling that it is going forwards to be supported, each time, by the next step, the steps here are made with the body weight remaining directly over the stepping, lifting foot. The loose, swaggering, lifting and swinging actions of shoulders, arms and hands are livelier than the small foot actions.

Movement Skills Training

1 In the 'Step and' a step forwards is taken on to the flat foot and the weight is transferred to it on the 'Step'. On the 'and', the other foot is placed beside the stepping foot, with the ball of the foot touching the floor, but not taking the body weight. 'Step and...; left and...; right and...'.

2 A three-step routine means that a different foot leads each time. The long first step is followed by two quick short steps. 'Left, right, left; right, left, right; slow, quick, quick; 1, 2, 3.'

3 In the 'Follow the Leader', ask the followers to look at and learn the foot movements first, and then look at and learn the upper body, arm and shoulder swinging gestures that will be 'partner originals' designed to contrast with the simpler, less expressive feet actions.

4 All can be encouraged to plan and perform bouncy, swinging, big, loose upper body, arm and shoulder movements to contrast with the smaller knee bouncing and steps.

Caribbean Maze Dance

An explanatory walk through of the maze behind the teacher will show the class what we mean by making and unravelling a circular maze. He or she emphasises 'If we make the maze travelling in an anti-clockwise circle that keeps becoming smaller and smaller, we then come out, still all following the same person, but in the opposite, clockwise direction. Keep walking. Keep thinking. Keep behind the one who started in front of you.' Teacher-led, whole class circle, and pupil-led, smaller circles then dance their mazes.

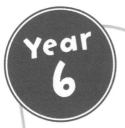

Year 6

Lesson Plan 12 • 30 minutes
June

Theme: *Responding to music.*

CD TRACK 27

Warm-up Activities
5 minutes

1 All crouch down in our large circle, bouncing on the spot.

2 Slowly rise up to standing and, on the spot, do easy steps and swings of free leg across standing leg.

3 Still facing the centre, do a side-to-side travel with a side, together, chasse action and hand-claps each time your feet come together. Do four side-to-side chasse steps to each side.

4 All travel into the centre and out again, tall with a good 'swagger' of upper body from side to side.

5 Half of class go into circle and out, while the other half go out backwards and in again. (Ask class to suggest contrasting actions for the back and forwards travels.)

6 Travel around in a circle, to right and to left, four steps each way.

Movement Skills Training
15 minutes

1 In your groups of four, travel to your agreed places for your own choice of activities. Decide your group shape – two facing two; all in a line; in a circle; staying on the spot; travelling all together; or one, then two, and so on; circling around, hands joined; wheeling around and back, one hand in, making a star.

2 Decide the footwork to be used, often the step-swing across.

3 Throughout, the travelling is slow, 'easy' and unhurried, often with an accompanying hand-clap or a bounce of the upper body.

Dance – In The Mood
10 minutes

Music: *In the Mood*, performed by Glenn Miller & his Orchestra (3 mins 27 secs)

1 From your separate groups, return, now, to the whole class circle, facing the centre, and stepping to right and to left, with hand-claps.

2 On the spot, place one elbow in the other hand. The wrist of the high, held hand rotates to right and to left.

3 Strong step-swings with opposite arm and leg swinging across.

4 Crouch, bouncing, slowly rising up to finish with a high spring and gesture of the arms at the end, 'Yeah!'

5 Brilliant. Now, let's dance it all the way through, starting in our big circle, crouching down.

Time	
0 secs	In a big circle, crouched, bouncing on the spot.
10 secs	Slow rise to standing.
15 secs	Easy steps with free leg swinging across standing leg.
28 secs	Side-to-side travel, facing centre, four chasse each way.
43 secs	All into centre and out again, with swagger of upper body.
56 secs	Half into circle and half out; then back to circle again.
1 min 6 secs	Travel in a circle, right and left, 4 counts each way.
1 min 36 secs	Own choices of group activities in groups of four.
2 mins 22 secs	All return to whole class circle, stepping right and left, with hand-claps.
2 mins 40 secs	On the spot, one elbow in the other hand, rotating.
3 mins 0 secs	Step-swings with opposite arm and leg swings across.
3 mins 15 secs	Crouch, bouncing, rising to high spring and 'Yeah!'

Dance

Teaching notes and NC guidance
Development over 4 lessons

Pupils should be taught to:

a respond to music. Pupils will be interested to learn that this is probably the best-known piece of big-band music from the era of big bands and ballroom dancing after the last war. In 'responding' to more than three minutes of music, it helps to have a start directed by the teacher, a middle planned by the groups, and an ending directed by the teacher.

b compose and control their movements by varying shape, size, level, direction, speed and tension. The groups of four will be asked to decide their group shape; actions and any travelling directions; and whether they will move with small, soft steps, big, swinging, strong leg and arm movements, or a mixture of the two.

Pupils should be able to show that they can respond imaginatively to the various challenges. The middle of the dance provides nearly one minute of pupil-centred, imaginative responding. For variety, the teacher might encourage different group alignments – a line, circle, square, wheel – but the content will be the result of group planning and group decision-making. Pupil response might include jiving by those who have attended Dance classes out of school.

Warm-up Activities

1 The circle is large with pupils well spaced apart from one another.

2 Staying on the same spot, they step on to one foot, taking all their weight, and swing the other leg across the supporting foot. 'Step and swing; right and left; left and swing.'

3 All stay in their circle positions for the four chasse 'step close' actions to each side. The teacher will decide 'Starting to your left, ready, go! Step, close and clap; left, close and clap; left, 2, 3; step, close and clap; now right, close, clap; to right, 2, 3.'

4 The easy, ordinary steps into the centre and out, are accompanied by the more exuberant, larger than life, swaggering upper body, shoulder and arm swings.

5 Number ones travel into the circle and back out while the number twos go backwards to start with, then forwards, to return to starting places.

6 Taking four counts each way, they travel to right and to left, staying in the big circle.

Movement Skills Training

1–3 After the totally teacher-directed start, the groups of four now go to the places provided by the teacher, to plan and practise the middle part of the lesson and the eventual dance. Because the steps and body movements will not be very different from group to group, the expression of their 'responding imaginatively' will be in their alignment; the ways they work to share the space; the patterns they follow as they travel; how they relate to one another; and what upper body actions they include to make their work more 'eye-catching'.

In The Mood Dance

A teacher-directed, simple addition becomes the start of the dance. After repeating all the work they have practised in the warm-up and the middle part of the lesson, the dance finishes with an on-the-spot, teacher-directed ending.

Lesson Plan 13 • 30 minutes
July

CD TRACK 28

Theme: *Responding imaginatively to music as members of a team.*

Warm-up Activities
5 minutes

1 Walk around freely, by yourself, to this well-known, slow, *Rock Around The Clock* music. Take one step to each count of the music, step and step, 1, 2, 3, 4.

2 The stepping is slow and you have plenty of time to add in big arm and shoulder swings from side to side for interest.

3 Face the front, feet still, doing big arm swings from side to side. Four swings standing; four with a bending of the knees; four with a stretching of the knees; and four standing.

4 Now, do eight lively hop-swings, where you step on to a foot, then hop and swing the opposite leg across the hopping one. Hop-swing; hop-swing; lively, lively; 5, 6, 7, keep going.

5 Well done. Walk again for eight counts, with free leg and opposite arm swinging straight forwards, then turn and do eight back again.

Movement Skills Training
10 minutes

1 In your groups of four, join hands in a small circle. Each chasse takes two counts of the music. Do five chasse in each direction.

2 Fours divide into two pairs who link right arms to do eight running steps to left, then to right with left arms linked. Your free arm is held high as you wave to the others. Go!

3 Well done. All stand ready to walk to the group lines starting place. Ready? Go! Into lines, face front.

4 Four arm swings, standing... knees bent... stretching... standing... eight hop swings to right.

5 Hop-swing, hop-swing, 3, 4, 5, 6, 7, to left; hop-swing, lively, 3, 4, 5, 6, 7, now walk right.

6 Walk, 2, 3, 4, 5, 6, 7, turn; walk back, 3, 4, 5, 6, make your circle.

7 Chasse left, 2, 3, 4, 5; chasse right, 2, 3, link arm with partner.

8 Quick running, elbows linked, 5, 6, 7, turn; quick running, wave other arm, 5, 6, 7, well done.

Dance — Rock 'n' Roll
15 minutes

Music: *(We're Gonna) Rock Around The Clock* **performed by Bill Haley and the Comets (2 mins 6 secs)**

1 In the middle of the dance, there are 30 seconds when your group of four will use imagination, please, and plan your very own actions. You can work together in a line; or moving, two by two, from your line; or in a rippling action down the line; or have pairs meeting and passing, under an arch; or one can perform on the spot with the others circling around .

2 For variety and contrast can you include at least two group actions?

3 To finish the dance, there will be 36 seconds during which all do the same movement, as at the start of the dance. All stand facing the same way, hands on the shoulders of the person in front of you.

4 Lets try the whole dance through.

Time	
0 secs	With the music, walk to places in lines.
10 secs	Face front, arm swings, standing; knees bending, knees stretching, standing.
20 secs	Hop-swing left and right, with arm and leg swings, now walk.
30 secs	Walk right, arm swings, 3, 4, 5, 6, 7, turn; left, left, swing arms, 5, 6, 7, into circle.
40 secs	Slow chasse to left and right, partners.
50 secs	Quick run, elbows joined, back again.
1 m	Own choices of group sequences.
1 m 30 secs	Bouncing lines, into big circle.
1 m 55 secs	Still in your circle, face the centre, holding partner with one hand while other hand waves to classmates.
2 m 6 secs	Music and dance end.

Dance

Teaching notes and NC guidance
Development over 3 lessons

Pupils should be able to show that they can:

a plan to respond imaginatively to challenges. To make the pupils' imaginative responses manageable, the teacher directs the start and the finish, and challenges the groups of four pupils to plan the middle of their dance.

b practise, improve and refine performance, and repeat a series of movements with increasing control and accuracy. We also want an enthusiastic, stylish and poised performance that is obviously being enjoyed enormously.

c make simple judgements about their own and others' performances and use this information to improve the quality. Appreciative, encouraging evaluation enhances the pleasure experienced when giving a performance.

Warm-up Activities

1–2 The stepping to the clear beat of the music is easy and encourages a good lifting of the knees on the steps, and a big, free shoulder and slightly-bent arm swings accompaniment. The arm and shoulder swings should encourage interesting individual responses.

3 The feet still, four part, a: b: c: a repeating pattern on the spot includes full arm swings standing; with knee bends; with knee stretches; standing.

4 The 'step-hop' involves a step on to the right foot followed by a hop on the right foot with a swing of the left leg across the right one. That swinging left leg then is stepped on and hopped on with an accompanying swing of right leg across to right. 'To right, hop-swing; to left, hop swing.'

5 The lively swing forwards with leading foot and opposite arm and shoulder is emphasised as they feel that they are reaching forwards with, for example, left leg and foot and right arm and shoulder.

Movement Skills Training

1 In the small circles of four, hands joined with well-bent arms, all chasse five times to each side.

2 Two pairs, with elbows joined, do eight running steps with high arm waving, clockwise, and then eight, anti-clockwise.

3 A revision of the free stepping start to the dance to make lines of four, all facing the front.

4 A revision of the four-part pattern of knees bending for 4, stretching for 4, and standing, all with full upper body, shoulder and arm swings.

5 A revision of the eight lively step-hops to the right and to the left.

6 A revision of the walking with opposite leg and arm swings, in both directions.

7 A revision of the chasse to left, 2, 3, 4, 5, and to right, 2, 3, 4, 5, in a circle, arms linked.

8 A revision of the elbows linked, running with other arm high waving, eight in each direction.

Rock 'n' Roll Dance

This dance has a teacher-directed start and finish and a pupil-planned middle to share out the work of being creative. The teacher's start gets the dance off to a whole class, united beginning. The teacher's ending brings the dance to a united, 'all together' climax. The 30-second middle of pupil-created group work, helped by the teacher's suggestions through '1–6' of this part of the lesson, gives this age group the opportunity to end their programme with something to be really proud of.

Games

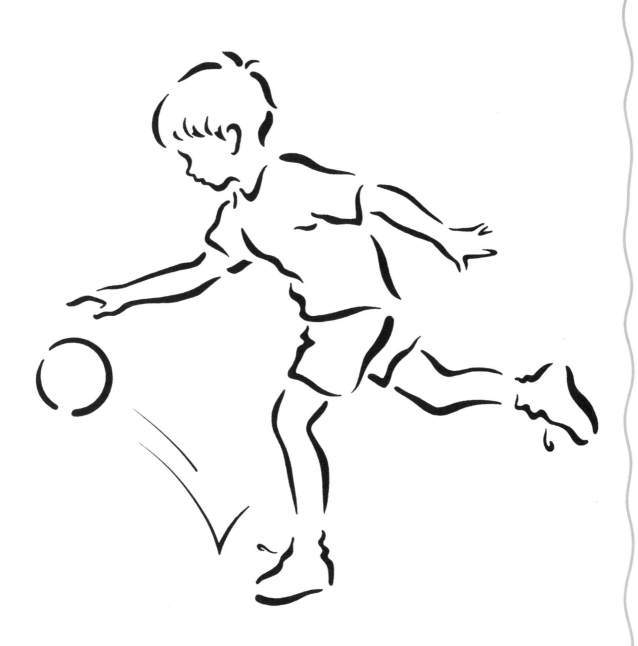

Introduction To Games

Individual and team games are part of our national heritage and an essential part of the physical education programme. Skills learned during games lend themselves to being practised away from school, alone or with friends or parents, and are the skills most likely to be used in participating in worthwhile physical and social activities long after leaving school – an important, long-term aim of physical education.

Vigorous, whole body activity in the fresh air promotes normal, healthy growth and physical development, stimulating the heart, lungs and big muscle groups, particularly the legs. Games lessons come nearest of all physical education activities to demonstrating what we understand by the expression 'children at play'. Pupils are involved in play-like, exciting, adventurous chasing and dodging as they try to outwit opponents in games and competitive activities. Such close, friendly 'combat' with others can help to compensate for the increasingly isolated, over-protected, self-absorbed nature of much of today's childhood.

All the lessons in this book are planned for the playground where most primary school games teaching now takes place. Precious time spent travelling to a field; the high cost of coach travel; a wet, muddy surface for much of the year; the need for expensive footwear; and a playing surface on which it is difficult to practise the variety of activities and small-sided games we need to offer, have all combined to make the school's own playground the preferred setting for the games programme.

Each rectangular third of the netball court is clearly marked with painted lines that should last for several years. These thirds are an ideal size for the three different games that are the climax of each lesson. It is recommended that schools have a line painted from end line to end line, in a different colour to ensure that the netball court is not affected. The extra line means that each rectangle is sub-divided into two halves. The line can be the centre for games across each third and a useful, definite marking for those games, where, for example, you may want to limit defenders or attackers to their own halves. The line can also be a 'net' for summer term games of short-tennis, quoits or volleyball.

The playground 'classroom' rectangle is essential because it contains the whole class in a limited space within which the teacher can see, and be easily seen and heard by, the whole class, and it prevents accidents by keeping the class well away from potential hazards such as concrete seats, hutted classrooms, fences or walls, all of which should be several metres outside the games rectangle.

Games will appeal to, and be very popular with the majority if: the pupils are always moving; the games are exciting; nobody is left doing nothing; they are fun to play; there is plenty of action; and if rules prevent quarrels, let the game run smoothly, let everyone have a turn, and prevent foul play.

The following monthly lesson plans and accompanying explanatory notes are designed to help teachers and schools with ideas for lessons that progress from month to month, and from year to year. Each lesson is repeated three or four times to allow plenty of time for planning, practising, repeating and improving. The plans also aim to provide a focus for staffroom togetherness and unity of purpose regarding the programme's aims, content, teaching methods, standards, and expectations of levels of achievement.

The Games Lesson Plan for Juniors – 30–45 minutes

All of the lessons that follow are designed for the school playground where most primary school games teaching takes place. Each rectangular third of the netball court is an ideal size for the three different, small-sided games or group practices which are the climax of each lesson.

Warm-up and Footwork Practices (4–6 minutes) start the lesson and aim to get the class quickly into action, and stimulate vigorous leg muscle activity which, in turn, stimulates the heart and lungs. Pupils enjoy practising running, jumping, chasing, dodging, marking, changing speed and direction, side-stepping, swerving and accelerating. Older juniors learn correct stopping and starting so that footwork rules in netball and basketball are understood. 'Faking' by moving head, shoulder or foot to one side, then suddenly moving the opposite way; sprint and change of direction dodges; and offensive and defensive footwork, used in 'one against one' dodges, are all practised.

Skills Practices (8–12 minutes) form the middle part of the lesson with the whole class using the same implement and practising the same skills so that the teaching and coaching applies to everyone. With younger, less experienced pupils, the practices include individual then partner practices of skills they might have performed before. They progress on to co-operative and competitive, partner and small group practices of skills already experienced to make practising more like the games situation.

Invent a Game or Skill Practice (3–5 minutes) provides pupils with the opportunity to plan a practice that further develops the skills featured in the middle part of the lesson, or to invent their own game complete with agreed rules and scoring systems.

Group Practices and Small-sided Games (15–22 minutes) can provide one of the most eagerly anticipated parts of all junior school physical education. They are the climax of the lesson and must be started promptly to allow their full time allocation. One of the three games or activities always includes use of the implement and skills practised in the middle part of the lesson. The three games or group practices take part in the thirds of the netball court. If a second court is available, it can be used for any activity that benefits from a bigger playing pitch. The three sets of implements to be used will have been placed adjacent to, but outside, the enclosed rectangles where they will be used.

The main organisational challenge is explaining and starting this final part of the lesson on the first day of a new series of lessons. At the start of the year, the six mixed teams or groups will have been chosen and given 'Your starting place for games and group activities.' If the teacher explains only one game at a time to the ten about to play it, the remaining twenty will be standing, losing heat and patience, and often becoming noisy and inattentive.

The answer is to have all three groups playing the same game or practice, one of the three to be introduced. Instructions about scoring, the main rules and method of re-starting after a score, will apply to all. The signal 'Start!' applies to everyone. When all three games are being played and are obviously understood, the teacher moves to and teaches one group its planned game or activity. When this group is going well, the teacher moves on to and teaches a second group its planned activity. The teacher then says 'Stop, everyone, and look at each of the two games or activities some of you have not seen yet.' Each new game or activity is demonstrated with an accompanying commentary from the teacher. The three groups then rotate on to their second activity, and finally to their third and last activity.

A Pattern for Teaching a Games Skill or Practice

Excellent lesson 'pace' is expressed in almost non-stop activity with no bad behaviour stoppages and no 'dead spots' caused by queues, over-long explanations or too many time-consuming demonstrations. The teaching of each of the skills combining to make a games lesson determines the quality of the lesson's pace – a main feature of an excellent physical education lesson.

A typical games lesson with its warm-up and footwork practices, skills practices, and small-sided group practices and games, will have about a dozen skills. Whatever the skill, there is a pattern for teaching it.

1   **Quickly into action**. In a few words, explain the task, and challenge the class to start. 'Can you stand, two big steps apart, and throw and catch the small ball to your partner for a two-handed catch?' If a short demonstration is needed, the teacher can work with a pupil who has been alerted. Class practice should start quickly after the five seconds it took the teacher to make the challenge.

2   **Emphasise the main teaching points, one at a time, while the class is working**. z A well-behaved class does not need to be stopped to listen to the next point. 'Hold both hands forward to show your partner where to aim.' 'Watch the ball into your cupped hands.'

3   **Identify and praise good work, while the class is working**. Comments are heard by all; remind the class of key points; and inspire the praised to even greater effort. 'Well done, Sarah and Daniel. You are throwing and catching at the right height and speed, and watching the ball into your hands.'

4   **Teach for individual improvement while class are working**. 'Liam, hold both hands forward to give Lucy a still target to aim at.' 'Chloe and Ben, stand closer. You are too far apart.'

5   **A demonstration can be used**, briefly, to show good quality or an example of what is required. 'Stop everyone, please, and watch how Ravinder and Michael let their hands "give" as they receive the ball, to stop it bouncing out again.' Less than twelve seconds later, all resume practising, understanding what 'giving hands' means.

6   **Very occasionally, to avoid taking too much activity time, a short demonstration can be followed by comments**. 'Stop and watch Leroy and Emily. Tell me what makes their throwing and catching so smooth and accurate.' The class watch about six throws and three or four comments are invited. For example, 'They are nicely balanced with one foot forward.' 'Their hands are well forward, to take the ball early, then give, smoothly and gently.'

7   **Thanks are given to performers and those making helpful comments**. Further practice takes place with reminders of the good things seen and commented on.

Progressing a Games Lesson over 4 or 5 Lessons

Gymnastic activities and dance lessons can begin at a simple level of performing the actions neatly, because they are natural and easy. The challenge for the teacher and class is then to plan and develop movement sequences that link these natural actions together, and refine them by adding 'movement elements' such as changes of speed, direction, shape and tension.

Developing a games lesson is different from the above because the eventual target is the mastery of the specific games skills included in the lesson. Such skills include:

○ good footwork used in stopping, starting, changing direction, chasing after and dodging away from other players

○ sending, receiving and travelling with a ball in invasion, striking/fielding and net games, and controlling other games implements such as skipping ropes, quoits, rackets, hoops and bean bags

○ inventing games with agreed rules in co-operation with a partner or small group. Fairness, safety, lots of action and an understanding of the need for rules are the intended outcomes

○ playing competitive games as individuals, with partners, and in small-sided games

○ understanding the skills and particular roles of players as they attack and defend in the three types of games.

Often the starting point, practising the new skill, is a problem, because controlling the implement is difficult. Balls, bats, hoops, skipping ropes, rackets, quoits and bean bags behave unpredictably and the teacher has to simplify the planned skills to enable pupils to succeed and progress in subsequent lessons. Reception class pupils, for example, might have to walk beside a partner, handing the bean bag to each other, before progressing to throwing and catching. In a Junior school, 2 versus 1 throwing and catching practice, the teacher can ask the defending pupil in the middle to be passive, with arms down at sides, not aiming to 'steal' the ball that is being passed, and only keeping between the two passing players to make them move sideways and forwards, into a good space to receive the ball.

The varied skills headings listed, fit neatly into both infant and junior games lessons, with their:

○ footwork practices

○ skills practices, which can include 'invent a game'

○ group practices and small-sided games, which can include 'invent a game' and challenges to suggest ways to improve a game with a new rule, other ways to score, or limits on player movement.

Step by step, revising the previous lesson's work, and introducing only one teaching point at a time, the teacher progresses one of the skills of the lesson, for example:

1   Try the slow overhead pull of the rope as it slides along the ground towards you.

2   Can you travel, running over the sliding rope, one foot after the other? Which is your leading leg?

3   On the spot, try a jump and bounce for each turn of the rope. (Slow '1 and, 2 and' skipping action.)

4   Try slow running over the rope. Use a small, turning wrist action with hands out wide at waist height.

5   Skip from space to space. Then show me skipping in each space.

6   On the spot, try the slow double beat and the quicker single beat. Then show me neat, non-stop skipping.

7   Pretend your group is on a stage, all doing your best skipping.

Invasion Games for Juniors – the Excitement of Competition

Outwitting one or more opponents – stages in progressing the level of competition

Stage 1 Offensive footwork practices without a ball – starting, stopping, changing direction, accelerating, sprinting, dodging, pivoting, feinting with head, foot or shoulder.

1 Jog, looking for spaces, when near others. Sprint suddenly when you have lots of room.

2 Run freely and change direction on 'Change!'

3 Practise side steps on to new line, still facing the same way.

Stage 2 Co-operative practices with a partner – dodges, direction changes, side steps, body fakes, changes of speed, and helpful comments from following, encouraging partner.

1 Follow your leader who will try dodges to lose you. Follower comments on the dodging.

2 Follow the leader who suddenly sprints to lose you, by speed and direction changes. Follower comments on which was the more successful – speed or direction changes.

3 Jog, side by side, at same speed. Leader does a sudden sprint to be free for a moment.

4 Partners face each other, one metre apart. Attacking partner progresses forward with small, rapid steps to try to make defender lose the 'in line' position between attacker and target line.

Stage 3 Competitive practices with a partner – gives 'attacking' player practice in checking the success of his or her repertoire of offensive dodges.

1 'Tag' where dodger tries to avoid being touched by chaser, who then becomes the dodger.

2 Dodge and Mark. Marker tries to stay within touching distance of dodger on teacher's 'Stop!'

3 One against one, across court, using body feints, plus direction and speed changes.

Stage 4 Offensive footwork practices with a partner, using a ball – trying to reach goal line with ball still in possession in dribbling games such as hockey, football or basketball. These little games need only a short stretch of line as a 'goal' with a 5 metre approach to this line.

1 Teacher allocates a number of minutes for each to attack from a start position 5 metres back. An attack ends when goal is scored, defender takes possession, or ball goes out of area.

2 In '3 lives' games, the same attacker starts three times, then changes roles.

Stage 5 Two against two practices with a ball – two kinds.

1 '3 lives', with same pair attacking three times from a 5 metre approach. After the three turns as attackers are used up, attackers become defenders.

2 End-to-end games across a third of the court with both teams trying to score. Passive defending, with the defending pair marking and keeping 'in line', but not tackling, encourages a flowing, enjoyable game for the less experienced.

Stage 6 Playing 3-, 4- or 5-a-side games – including scaled-down netball, hockey, basketball, football, handball, rugby touch, and created games such as heading ball, skittleball and hoop ball.

1 Attackers ideally understand – 'Pass and move!' 'Give and go to be available!'

2 A named team-mate moves to opponents' line as 'target player' to receive or give passes.

3 'Fast break' every time your team steals possession when none of your team is marked.

National Curriculum Requirements for Games – Key Stage 2: the Main Features

'The government believes that two hours of physical activity a week, including the National Curriculum for Physical Education and extra-curricular activities, should be an aspiration for all schools. This applies to all key stages.'

Programme of study Pupils should be taught to:

a play and make up small-sided and modified competitive net, striking/fielding and invasion games

b use skills and tactics and apply basic principles suitable for attacking and defending

c work with others to organise and keep the games going.

Attainment target Pupils should be able to demonstrate that they can:

a select and use skills, actions and ideas appropriately, applying them with co-ordination and control

b when performing, draw on what they know about tactics and strategy

c compare and comment on skills and ideas used in own work by modifying and refining skills and techniques.

Main NC headings when considering progression and expectation

Planning: Performing and participating in a thoughtful, well-organised way is the result of good planning, which takes place before and during performance. Subsequent performances will be influenced by the planning that also takes place after reflecting on the success or otherwise of the activity. Where planning standards are considered to be satisfactory, there is evidence of: (a) thinking ahead; (b) good judgements and decisions; (c) good understanding; (d) originality; (e) consideration for others; (f) positive qualities such as enthusiasm, whole-heartedness and the capacity for working and practising hard to achieve.

Performing and improving performance: We are fortunate in Physical Education because of the visual nature of the activities. It is easy to see, note and remember how pupils perform, demonstrating skill and versatility. Where standards of performing are satisfactory there is evidence of: (a) neatness, accuracy and 'correctness'; (b) skilfulness and versatility; (c) the ability to remember and repeat; (d) safe, successful outcomes; (e) originality of solutions; (f) ability to do more than one thing at a time, linking a series of actions with increasing fluency, accuracy, control and skill; (g) ability to make sudden adjustments as needed; (h) pleasure from participation; (i) a clear understanding of what was required.

Evaluating/reflecting: Evaluation is intended to inform further planning and preparation by helping both performers and spectators with guidance and ideas for altering, adapting, extending and improving performances. Where standards in evaluating are satisfactory, pupils are able to: (a) observe accurately; (b) identify the parts of a performance that they liked; (c) pick out the main features being demonstrated; (d) make comparisons between two performances; (e) reflect on the accuracy of the work; (f) comment on the quality of the movement, using simple terms; (g) suggest ways in which the work might be improved; (h) express pleasure in a performance.

Year 6 Games Programme

Pupils should be able to:

Autumn	Spring	Summer
1 Dress sensibly from safety and hygiene points of view.	**1** Achieve a high level of physical activity in all lessons and understand its effect on the body.	**1** Perform skills of net and striking/fielding games with increasing control and confidence.
2 Respond readily to sensible rules and instructions.	**2** Improve skills of sending, receiving and travelling with a ball, using hands, feet and stick.	**2** Play small-sided versions of recognised games – cricket, tennis, rounders, volleyball, stoolball.
3 Respond quickly to others' actions, planning and applying quick decision-making.	**3** Sustain energetic activity to maintain winter warmth.	**3** Be aware of varying roles and skills as a member of a team – bat, bowl, field, keep wicket, serve, backhand, forehand, volley.
4 Understand and apply the footwork rule in games.	**4** Respond quickly to a changing environment and adjust to other people's actions.	**4** Improve and repeat longer, more complex sequences – rallies in tennis and volleyball; flowing bowling, batting, fielding and throwing in, in cricket.
5 Develop versatility and variety in ways of travelling with, sending and receiving a ball.	**5** Experience small-sided versions of recognised games – football, netball, basketball, hockey, rugby.	**5** Show awareness of simple court positions, e.g. return to centre after each stroke.
6 Use own 'invented games' to apply skills learned in lesson.	**6** Plan extra ways to score to make games more interesting. 'Score either in hoop, one point, or on line, two points.'	**6** Demonstrate capacity, as a class, to organise selves and get games started quickly.
7 Improve and use effective footwork – pivoting, changing speed and direction, dodging.	**7** Use attacking principles, e.g. varied team shapes, diamond 1:2:1 or square 2:2, to spread defence to make space.	**7** Demonstrate accurate bowling, controlled batting, and quick-off-the-mark fielding and quick throwing in.
8 Understand common skills in attack and defence, e.g. 'shape' game in attack to make space; switch quickly from defence to attack; fast break, passing often, dribbling seldom; cover a defending partner.	**8** Understand common skills and principles in defence, e.g. marking opponent with or without ball, full court or half court, 1-on-1 defence.	**8** Plan, perform and reflect on the success of own, created games, and suggest ways to improve them.
9 Show good sporting behaviour.	**9** Learn and apply the specific rules of different games.	**9** Work harder, enthusiastically, for longer, in a focused way with poise, control and adaptability.
10 Make positive contributions to a group in co-operative and competitive situations.	**10** Suggest ways to improve a performance by others.	
11 Plan and use simple tactics and judge their success.		

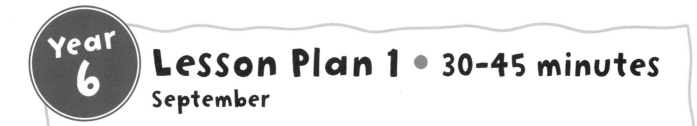

Year 6

Lesson Plan 1 • 30-45 minutes
September

Warm-up and Footwork Practices
4—6 minutes

1 Run quietly and well, tall and relaxed, keeping away from all others. When I call 'Stop!' check to see that you are not near anyone. Keep looking for spaces and running into them.

2 Free-and-caught. 6 chasers wearing coloured bands try to touch and catch others who then stand still with both hands on top of head. Those caught can be freed by others not caught touching them on the elbow.

Skills Practices: with large balls
8—12 minutes

Partner practices

1 Revise chest, bounce and overhead passing at 3 metres apart and move into a new space for the return pass.

2 Shadow dribble as in basketball. Changes of hand, speed, height for variety.

3 Juggle with hand, foot, head or thigh to strike ball upwards, and allow 1 bounce only between touches. What is your best score?

Invent a Game or Practice in 2s
3—5 minutes

Can you invent a game with one ball and 3–4 metres of a line? Include dodging, travelling with ball. (For example, in rugby, basketball or football fashion, can one player score by placing ball on line guarded by the other player?)

Group Practices and Small-sided Games
15—22 minutes

Dribbling-tag

Large ball each. Dribble basketball fashion, ball in control (illustrated). Touch others to score. Think of a rule to make game more interesting.

Bench-ball

4 or 5 a side. Pass to team-mate on chalk 'bench' to score. No-one else may go on bench. Change bench-catcher often, particularly on cold days.

2 half-pitch games of ground-level football

Large, flattish ball among 4. B v C v D, trying to score past A, the goalkeeper. Scorer becomes goalkeeper. At least 2 dribbling touches before shooting.

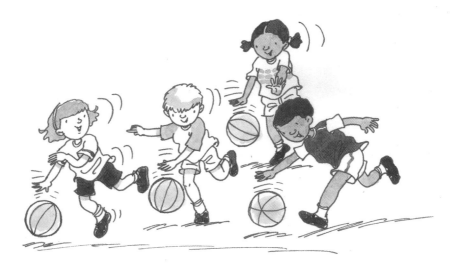

Games

Teaching notes and NC guidance
Development over 4–5 lessons

Lesson's main emphases:

a Improving the skills of sending, receiving and travelling with a ball in invasion games.

b Ensuring that September is used to re-establish the traditions which are essential for a successful and enjoyable Games programme – working quietly, but vigorously; responding to instructions immediately; and unselfishly sharing space.

Equipment: 15 large balls; 2 flattish balls for football and 4 cones for goals; playground chalk to mark 'bench'.

Warm-up and Footwork Practices

1 Insist on silent running in good style with heels and knees lifting. Run along straight lines, not in a circle all following each other. 'Stop!' is an exercise in gaining an immediate response. Praise the quick responders and rebuke others who need to smarten up.

2 In free-and-caught, stop the game every 12 seconds or so, to establish control and check the success of the chasers. Insist on 'gentle touches only when catching, with no dangerous pushing.'

Skills Practices: with large balls

Partner practices

1 The teacher has the right to expect the skills of passing, catching and dribbling to be done well after several years of being practised. 'Court circulation' and the way the children move after passing now become the main teaching points. We move to find a space to receive a return pass. We move to take a pass on the move when it is passed to one side or ahead of us. We move away from the action sometimes to leave more room for others in our team to do things, unhindered by those standing around.

2 With a well-spread hand, use your wrist, not elbow or shoulder, as the moving part to bounce the ball. Crouch slightly, down nearer the ball, with bent knees for closer control but a straight back to be able to see around you.

3 Ball is being sent by many body parts, with one bounce in between. Player must keep 'on toes' to be able to move quickly to be nicely balanced for next strike up.

Invent a Game or Practice in 2s

Both need to agree the nature of the game; how to score fairly; how and where to re-start after a goal; when to change roles; and the one main rule to make the game fair.

Group Practices and Small-sided Games

Dribbling-tag

In dribbling-tag, use low dribbling stance with hips and knees well bent, back straight, head up. To add interest, rule that a player on a line is 'safe', but must keep dribbling.

Bench-ball

In bench-ball, where lots of opponents may be crowding in front of catcher, encourage chest, bounce and overhead passes, with good fakes to mislead the marking opponents.

2 half-pitch games of ground-level football

Careful, not too hard, low shots at goal, so ball not forever being lost. All think of ways to give player with ball more time and space.

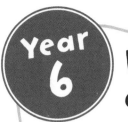

Year 6

Lesson Plan 2 • 30–45 minutes
October

Warm-up and Footwork Practices
4–6 minutes

1   Run, jump, land, 1, 2. Do not move back foot, which landed first. Pivot on it, with moving front foot looking for a space. Then run, jump, land, 1, 2, pivot, again.

2   Long-line tag. Start with 4 couples as chasers with hands joined. When caught by a couple, join the line and continue chasing. Last caught is winner.

Skills Practices: with large balls
8–12 minutes

Partner practices

1   Throw to partner who runs, jumps to catch ball above head, lands one foot in front of other, 1, 2, then pivots on rear foot and throws high pass to partner now running to jump to receive return pass.

2   Stand 2 metres apart, throw for partner to head back for you to catch. Eyes on ball, use forehead. Place one foot in front of the other for good balance. Change after 6 headers.

Invent a Game or Practice in 2s
3–5 minutes

Invent a game with one ball and part (3–4 metres) of a line. Throw, catch and/or head. (For example, heading-tennis over the line, with or against your partner.)

Group Practices and Small-sided Games
15–22 minutes

Mini-basketball

Netball apparatus, 4 or 5 a side. Dribbling permitted but 'pass and run' for more open, exciting game. 1 point for near miss if ball hits basket, 2 for a score. Apparatus in 2 metres from end line so ball not always going 'out' after a shot.

Heading-ball

4 or 5 a side, large foam ball. Score if ball headed over opponents' end line after pass from team-mate (illustrated). Good attack tactic to have one player near opponents' line for easy pass back to team-mate running forwards for header at goal.

Hockey

2 a side, half-pitch, '3 lives' games. Attackers start from centre and try to outwit and score against defenders. When a team has won or intercepted ball 3 times (lives), teams change places and duties.

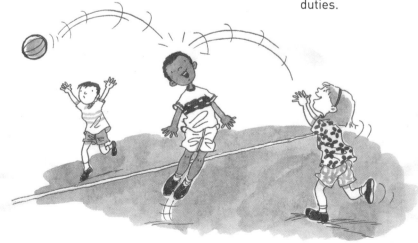

Games

Teaching notes and NC guidance
Development over 4–5 lessons

Lesson's main emphases:

a The NC requirements to understand and play small-sided versions of recognised games, and to make appropriate decisions quickly and plan their responses.

b Remembering that the most important and climactic part of the lesson is the last part, the group practices and small-sided games. To ensure that this part is never cut short, leading to 3 very short, therefore frustrating games, the teacher needs to be aware that the command to 'Begin!' the games must be given at least 15 or 22 minutes (short or long lesson) before the command 'Stop everyone!', when equipment is collected and the lesson ended. This tradition is as important as those emphasised in the last lesson.

Equipment: 15 large balls; 1 large foam ball; 10 hockey sticks and 2 balls.

Warm-up and Footwork Practices

1 Pivoting around on your rear foot is allowed in netball and basketball. Jump and land, calling out '1, 2' as each foot lands. The one to land first is fixed as the pivot foot. Rotate on the ball of this foot with heel lifted. Front foot does the moving, 'looking' for a partner to pass to. A pivot can also be used as a fake to evade a close marking opponent.

2 Start with 2 or 3 quartets as chasers, possibly with 1 working in each third of the court.

Skills Practices: with large balls

Partner practices

1 The point of pivoting, to land legally and to be mobile on the spot, will become obvious in the partner practice, which emphasises that Year 6 games players are expected to be mobile before and after receiving passes.

2 In the heading practice, 'Keep your eyes open and aim your header at your partner's hands.' Eyes shut and passively letting ball hit forehead are the usual faults.

Invent a Game or Practice in 2s

The line can be the goal an attacker has to throw, roll, kick, bounce, carry or head the ball across. The line can also be a net for heading/football/tennis over.

Group Practices and Small-sided Games

Mini-basketball

Ask players to shape the game when they are attacking. Opponents should be marking '1 on 1', and a diamond shape, for example, makes an open formation and easier passing, particularly if the rear court guard and their markers have to stay in one half.

Heading-ball

With a diamond attacking formation in heading-ball, the target player at front of diamond can head for goal, or catch and pivot to look for a running team-mate to whom to pass.

Hockey

One hockey rule which might help to make game more enjoyable is 'No tackling by defender. Confront the player with the ball and they must pass it.' Goal can be a hit between cones 3 metres apart.

Lesson Plan 3 • 30-45 minutes
November

Warm-up and Footwork Practices
4—6 minutes

1   Free running over whole court. Jog or sprint as space permits. To sprint, increase heel and knee lift, forwards lean of body. Use short, rapid arm movements.

2   Couples-tag. 3 couples start as chasers, hands joined. When one of couple touches a dodger, the dodger and that chaser change places.

Skills Practices: with hockey sticks and balls
8—12 minutes

Partner practices

1   Shadow dribbling: leader makes 6 touches of ball then swaps with following partner, who repeats leader's sequence. Gentle taps, stick near ground in front of player.

2   Push pass across 4 or 5 metres. Watch approaching ball carefully. Note to which side partner is running into a space. Receive ball, pass to partner's new position, then move for return pass into good open space.

Invent a Game or Practice in 2s
3—5 minutes

Invent a practice with one ball to develop dribbling and/or passing and receiving. (For example, 10 metres apart, one dribbles ball up to and around partner and returns to starting place. Ball pushed to partner who repeats. Coach each other for improvement.)

Group Practices and Small-sided Games
15—22 minutes

Hockey

2 v 2, 2 games. Dribblers or passers aim to arrive on, or pass ball to partner to finish on, opponents' goal line, ball in control under stick (illustrated).

Junior-netball

4 or 5 a side, all may score. Left- and right-side defenders and attackers keep to own sides of court for 'open' game and better visibility for marking when opponent has ball.

New-image rugby

4 or 5 a side, 4-person scrums. Place ball down on opponents' goal line to score. If touched on hips by opponent's two hands, pass forwards in own half, sideways or backwards in opponents'. Run fast and straight with ball.

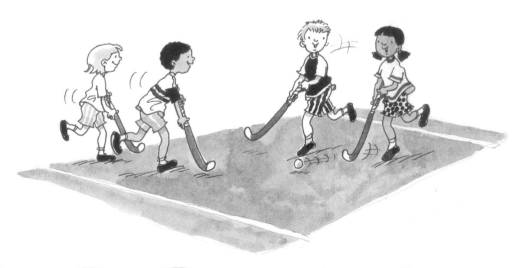

Games

Teaching notes and NC guidance
Development over 4–5 lessons

Lesson's main emphases:

a The NC requirements to explore and understand common skills and principles, including attack and defence in invasion games, and to play fairly, compete honestly and demonstrate good sporting behaviour.

b Knowing and sticking to team positions and marking an opponent closely. These are the two greatest contributors to making our games start to look more advanced and expert. The 'bees all around the honey pot' situation, typical of games in a small area, can only be changed when forwards, centres and defenders understand their positions and try to operate in those areas, instead of all chasing after the ball, all the time. If your opponent marks and stays with you, when your team has possession, you can take him away from the action to give team-mates more space.

Equipment: 30 hockey sticks and small balls; 1 large ball; 1 rugby ball.

Warm-up and Footwork Practices

As they warm up, running freely, using the whole area, it is a good idea to stop the class occasionally, ask them all to stand in a space as far away from others as possible, and observe the vast number of open spaces which you hope they will strive to create in their games. Only good positioning and pulling defenders into the shape you wish can produce this.

Skills Practices: with hockey sticks and balls

Partner practices

1 Dribbling should now include reverse stick work, toe down and flat surface to right, as well as normal toe-up dribbling, face of stick to left. Stick turn created by left hand turning the stick inside loose, sleeve-like, right-hand grip.

2 The push, made by placing stick next to ball and pushing, makes no sound and follows through low in front. Stick never goes behind you where it might strike someone.

Invent a Game or Practice in 2s

One partner gives the other a commentary of dribbling actions: 'straight; zigzag to left and right; then short push forwards to dribble around me; now pass to me for my turn.'

Group practices and Small-sided Games

Hockey

In 2-versus-2 hockey across half of one third of the court, encourage children to agree rules to help game flow more smoothly, for example defenders do not tackle, they confront to make attacker pass, and might stay in own half to help attack.

Junior-netball

In netball, 'pivot often to look for running partner; to stop, nicely in balance; to fake marking opponent to go wrong way.'

New-image rugby

In new-image rugby we can go on to a 4-person scrum after a forward pass in opponents' half. 'Scrum half' places ball for team-mate in scrum to hook back. Rest of scrum passive.

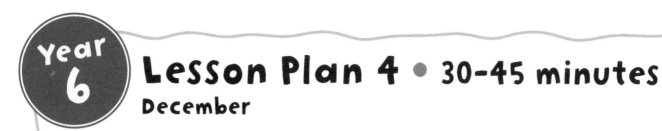

Lesson Plan 4 • 30-45 minutes
December

Warm-up and Footwork Practices
4—6 minutes

1   All run to end of court then return using 'boxer's shuffle' sideways, backwards to starting line, to practise defensive footwork. Feet apart, hips low, weight forwards.

2   Dodge and mark across court, 1 versus 1, side line to side line. Marker moving backwards tries to stop partner running past him to cross the side line. Keep rotating duties.

Skills Practices: with rugby balls or large balls
8—12 minutes

Small group practices

1   4s, one ball, half or third of court. Move, interpass to team-mate running to receive. Use corners and do not always move when others running into spaces.

2   3 versus 1 in small area, team passing. 3 passes = a goal. Change '1' often. Stress 'pass and move': having passed, move into a space, ready to receive.

Invent a Game or Practice in 4s
3—5 minutes

Invent a game to develop passing, catching, running into spaces. (For example, in a square facing inwards, 6 metres apart, A passes to B, follows ball to touch B's corner and back to own place. B passes to C, follows and returns, etc.)

Group Practices and Small-sided Games
15—22 minutes

New-image rugby

4/5 a side, 4-person scrums, line-outs. Place ball down over opponents' line to score. Pass when hip tackled by opponent's 2 hands. Forward pass in own half, sideways or backwards only in opponents'. Agree positions to shape and space team.

Floor-football

4/5 a side with flattish ball. Arrive on opponents' end line, ball under foot, to score. Ball below knee height. Left/right attackers or defenders on own sides of court so that it is easy to see who to work against or to mark. Receive; find team-mate; pass; move.

Change-bench-ball

4/5 a side. Goal when team-mate on bench catches your pass and throws to another on court before leaving bench. You become new bench-catcher. Vary passes to bench-catcher. Fakes mislead opponents.

Games

Teaching notes and NC guidance
Development over 4–5 lessons

Lesson's main emphases:

a The NC requirement to plan and make up their own games, and to practise, refine and improve performance.

b Emphasising the '1-on-1' marking as an important feature of our lesson to make the physical demands even greater, help to maintain mid-winter warmth, and make the games start to look more like end of Key Stage 2 standard – understanding offence and defence; using simple tactics; understanding roles as team members.

Equipment: 8 large or rugby balls; 1 flattish large ball for football; 1 large ball and playground chalk for drawing 'benches' in bench-ball.

Warm-up and Footwork Practices

1 Class can mirror teacher in the 'boxer's shuffle' defensive footwork practice, moving backwards against an imaginary opponent.

2 In 1-versus-1, cross-court dodge-and-mark to practise defensive footwork, ask attackers not to sprint past defenders. They should use careful, varied dodges, changing speed or direction and using head, foot and shoulder fakes.

Skills Practices: with rugby balls or large balls

Small group practices

1 Only pass to a moving player with a well-aimed pass ahead of him. Others can help by keeping out of the way and leaving space for the running player.

2 To give the '1' a chance, there is no running with the ball, as is normal in rugby.

Invent a Game or Practice in 4s

The main feature to practise is the running into spaces. If running to receive a pass, the space can be in front, behind or to either side of you, particularly if it follows a successful dummy or fake, deceptive move to take your opponent another way.

Group Practices and Small-sided Games

New-image rugby

In new-image rugby, we now have 4-person scrums when ball is wrongly passed forwards in opponents' half, and 4-person lineouts when ball goes over a side line. Non-offending team put ball in and only they are allowed to play the ball.

Floor-football

Floor-football is spoiled by all players wanting the ball and all being in a tiny area, usually with no possibility of open play or good passing movements. Enlist suggestions of class to make game more open and enjoyable by limiting some players to certain parts of the court. If defenders stay in own half; if defenders do not tackle team in its own half; if attackers have 1 'free' pass that is not intercepted, for example, the game will improve for everyone.

Change-bench-ball

Change-bench-ball demands quick decision-making by the scoring team. Defending team have to decide 'Who am I marking now?'

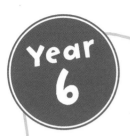
Lesson Plan 5 • 30-45 minutes
January

Warm-up and Footwork Practices
4—6 minutes

1 Run around quietly with tall, relaxed action, and practise side steps or changes of direction to avoid others coming straight towards you.

2 Chain-tag. 3 or 4 couples are chasers. When caught, join the chain. When it grows to 4, split into 2 chains and continue to chase. Last one caught wins.

Skills Practices: with large balls
6—10 minutes

Partner practices

1 3 metres apart, show me 2-handed chest and bounce passes to your partner after making a fake pass in other direction. Move to new space for return pass.

2 Follow-the-leader, football dribbling for 6 touches. Vary feet, speed, direction, parts of feet. Following partner observes, remembers sequence and repeats it on 'Change!'

Invent a Game or Practice in 4s
4—6 minutes

Can you 4 invent a game or practice to develop hand or foot control with 2 balls? (For example, while 2 count their rapid passes at 3 metres apart, the other 2 dribble around them, 1 at a time. Change duties and see which pair makes more passes.)

Group Practices and Small-sided Games
16—23 minutes

Floor-football

4 or 5 a side with flattish ball. Score by arriving, ball in control, on opponents' goal line. Ball below knee height. 2 defenders stay in own half. Left/right side attackers and defenders play on own sides for 'open' play. 'Pass often, move to new space to help.'

Mini-basketball

4 or 5 a side, netball apparatus. 1 target player stays near opponents' basket when his team has ball, to receive pass for easy shot at goal or pass back to team-mate in position to shoot (illustrated). Agree how to restart after goal and whether to allow dribbling.

Playground-hockey

4 or 5 a side, push-pass only. Scoring push in front half of opponents' court only. No hitting. Shape team into left- and right-side attackers and defenders for better spacing. Agree 1 rule to help game, for example 1 v 1 only.

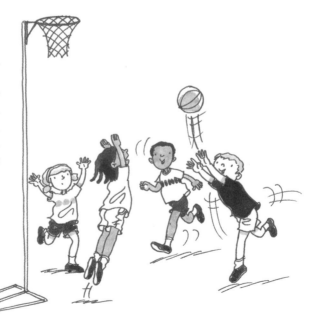

Games

Teaching notes and NC guidance
Development over 4–5 lessons

Lesson's main emphases:

The NC places a very big emphasis on planning, performing and reflecting in Physical Education. The doing or performing, particularly in cold January, should be uppermost in the teacher's intentions anyway. The planning is straightforward and should be being asked for continually throughout the lesson. The challenging words 'Can you...?' or 'Show me...' call for planning to answer the tasks. For example, 'Can you plan to include changes of feet, speed or direction in your dribbling sequence where your partner is following?' and 'In attack in your three games, can you plan to move into a space every time you have passed the ball?' Team-mates with the ball then know that at least one of their team is going to try hard to be available for the next pass. Other team-mates can help by keeping out of the way and pulling their defender out of the way.

Reflection/evaluation, usually after a demonstration by an individual, a pair or a group, is not so easy in mid-winter when we want to keep inactive, stationary moments to an absolute minimum. To enable almost non-stop activity from beginning to climactic, busy, exciting end of the lesson, it is recommended that we ask for very few comments immediately after the demonstration and continue the reflecting in class after the lesson.

Teacher questioning while the activities are continuing might inspire all to reflect more while working. For example, 'While you are defending in your three games, can you feel where your body weight should be while you are 'boxer's shuffling' backwards?' (Weight should be forwards on balls of feet, not back.)

Reflection leads to planning and adapting in a more focused way and should lead to better, more efficient and correct performing.

The teacher should be planning to keep the class active for the maximum number of minutes out of the 30 or 45 so that when the children reflect on their January Games lesson, they are agreed that they performed almost non-stop, kept warm and had three good-length games to finish with.

Equipment: 15 large balls; 10 hockey sticks and 1 ball.

Group Practices and Small-sided Games

Floor-football

The difficulty in controlling the lively ball and evading the very close-marking opponents makes the game difficult for the attacking team. If necessary, for a more enjoyable attacking game, place limits on the defenders. For example, no tackling in a team's own half; or allow one unhindered pass before you may tackle; or only one defender ever allowed to tackle one attacker.

Mini-basketball

If necessary, for a more flowing, enjoyable attacking game, leave the target player unmarked to encourage a quick advance of the ball, with minimum dribbling or delay, to the opponents' end of the court. The target player, with his back to the basket, must be encouraged to keep moving into good spaces to receive a chest, bounce or overhead pass.

Playground-hockey

In hockey, encourage the attackers to shape the game with some keeping well away, to provide space. Insist on defenders marking own opponents (i.e. being shaped and spread out by attackers).

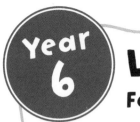

Lesson Plan 6 • 30-45 minutes
February

Warm-up and Footwork Practices
4–6 minutes

1   Follow-the-leader, trying to include at least three different leg activities you can practise, improve and perform together.

2   Dodge-and-mark in 2s. On 'Stop!' both freeze. Dodger clear of marker's reach or marker able to touch dodger wins. Change duties.

Skills Practices: with hockey sticks and balls
6–8 minutes

Partner practices

1   Shadow dribble, both with ball. Leader does easy left and harder right turn where feet move ahead of ball so it is behind as you overtake it.

2   Right-side dodge. Practise dribbling up to your partner, who is facing you. Push ball past non-stick side of partner, run past partner by going to own left. Practice 6 times and change.

Invent a Game
4–6 minutes

Invent a 2 v 2 game to develop dribbling and dodging, in half of third of court, for example 'three lives', half-pitch game. Attacking pair have ball. Defenders, one on goal line, one on court, try to steal ball three times. Score by arriving on line, ball in control under stick. Change over.

Group Practices and Small-sided Games
16–25 minutes

Playground-hockey

4 or 5 a side. In own half quick pass to team-mate to clear ball from near own goal. In opponents' half outwit opponents with right-side dodge or good dribble. Scoring pass from within opponents' half only.

New-image rugby

4 or 5 a-side, 4-person scrums. Score by placing ball down behind opponents' goal line. Pass when touched on hips by opponents' 2 hands. No forward passing. Fakes to fool opponents. In 4-person scrum, scrum half puts ball by right foot of far team-mate, the only one who may hook ball back.

Free-netball

4 or 5 a side with no scoring restrictions. Forwards and defenders all mark opponent with ball. When team-mate has ball, dodge to lose marker long enough to receive pass. Think of ways to score in addition to netball ring, for example target hoops at ends.

Games

Teaching notes and NC guidance
Development over 4–5 lessons

Lesson's main emphases:

a   The NC requirements to sustain energetic activity and show understanding of what is happening to their bodies while exercising, and to explore and understand common skills and principles, including attack and defence, in invasion games.

b   Emphasising that the lesson is full of examples of players being in close proximity to other players, dodging, shadowing and marking. In our games let us try the fast break as an attacking tactic, to travel from one end to the other at full speed before the opposing defenders. 'Get there fastest with the mostest!' is an American expression for a main tactic from the world of professional basketball.

It is essential for the whole team to be thinking 'fast break' so that when they suddenly steal the ball or it is their throw-in after a goal, the ball is passed rapidly down court to fast breaking players, all looking for a pass in an open space. Three such passes can send the ball to the opposite end before the opponents, running backwards, arrive there.

   At the moment of a 'change of possession', when team A steal or intercept the ball from team B, all team A members are unmarked because team B had been trying to get away from team A. At that moment, team A should take advantage of not being marked to 'fast break!' before team B pick up and mark their opponents again.

   During the 'fast break' learning period, the class can be asked to co-operate in helping to produce good fast breaks by being quite passive in defence during the first few seconds of an attempted fast break, possibly allowing two or three passes to advance unimpeded.

   Players knowing their respective positions – left- or right-side attack or defence, or centre – is essential to good fast breaking progress down the court. Good '1-on-1' marking is equally important so that the game is being shaped by the attacking players to allow room for good individual attacking to be practised.

Equipment: 30 hockey sticks and 15 small balls; 1 rugby ball; 1 large ball and netball apparatus.

Group Practices and Small-sided Games

Playground-hockey

Team with ball thinks 'minimum dribbling in own half; much first time passing to "break" quickly; shape game in opponents' half to create spaces for easy passing or individual dribble to score.'

New-image rugby

In new-image rugby, a 4-person scrum is awarded to the non-offending team after a forward pass anywhere now. Ball thrown in to foot of far team-mate in scrum, the only player allowed to strike the ball back from scrum.

Free-netball

Occasionally, in this and the other two games, the teacher should call 'Stop!' to check that defenders are marking their own opponents and that attackers are trying to shape the game.

Lesson Plan 7 • 30-45 minutes
March

Warm-up and Footwork Practices
4—6 minutes

1   Steady run beside partner. Now 'sprint dodge' ahead for a moment, then slow down to side-by-side run again. Repeat. Change duties.

2   10-points tag. All start with 10 points. Lose 1 each time touched. Teacher checks who has most points left and who caught most.

Skills Practices: with rugby balls and large balls
8—12 minutes

Small group practices

1   4s, file pass and follow, rugby passing. A passes to B and runs to end of opposite line, B to C, then runs to end of opposite line. How many passes by your team in 30 seconds?

2   4s, pick up, put down. One picks ball up on line, runs to put it down after 3 metres, then runs to opposite end. Others in turn pick same ball up and put down after 3 metres.

Invent a Skills Practice in 4s
3—5 minutes

Invent a run, pass, touch-down practice with 2 balls. (For example, run pass to partner in small part of third of court. On 'Change!', all balls touched down, find new partner and ball, start again.)

Group Practices and Small-sided Games
15—22 minutes

New-image rugby

4 or 5 a side. Score by placing ball down over opponents' line. Re-start with back pass at centre. No forward passing. Pass after two-hand touch on hips by opponent. Devise extra ways to score, for example target hoops at corners to bounce ball in.

Handball

4 or 5 a side. Score by throwing ball from outside goal semi-circle into goal. Goalkeeper only allowed in scoring area (illustrated). Challenge teams to suggest other ways to score, for example knock down a goalskittle.

2 versus 2, half-pitch, '3 lives' games

Choice of football, netball, basketball, hockey, rugby-touch or heading-ball. After defenders make 3 scores or interceptions change over duties.

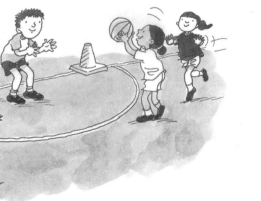

Teaching notes and NC guidance
Development over 4–5 lessons

Lesson's main emphases:

a The NC requirement to understand, make up and play small-sided versions of recognised competitive games.

b Encouraging the class to think beyond the limited, traditional ways of scoring in running/invasion games so that the games become more exciting, scoring increases and more children go home saying 'I scored today!' For example, 1 point might be awarded in rugby for a score in a hoop. 2 points can be scored by a traditional try. In handball, 2 points for a ball through the goal, 1 point for a ball bounced into a hoop, also in the scoring area. 1 point for a near miss, hitting ring in netball or basketball, 2 points for a shot passing through the hoop.

Equipment: 8 rugby or large balls; 1 large ball for handball; and large balls, hockey sticks and balls for the choice of games in 2 versus 2, '3 lives' games; netball apparatus.

Warm-up and Footwork Practices

1 A sprint dodge is a sudden and excellent way to shake free of a close-marking opponent, momentarily, to receive a pass.

2 In 10-points tag, ask class to plan ways of dodging others, and to recognise what they (or other impressive dodgers) are doing. Sprint dodges; head, foot and shoulder fakes; direction changes.

Skills Practices: with rugby or large balls

Small group practices

1 4s, file pass and follow, should build up to a pass each second. 'And 1, and 2...' where 'and' is the pass, and the number is the run by passer.

2 The pick-up, put-down relay, practising gathering and the act of scoring, is played across a 12-metre area. Remember to score by a two-hand touch down on top of the ball, not a throw down.

Invent a Skills Practice in 4s

For example, three pass one ball, dodging fourth with own ball with which he tries to touch a ball-handler. When he succeeds, both balls are touched down on ground. Caught player picks up a ball to become new chaser, and one of the other three picks up other to re-start.

Group Practices and Small-sided Games

New-image rugby

A re-start with pass back at centre after rugby try means no forward passing henceforth. 4-person scrum after a pass forwards, and 4-person line-out after the ball goes out of play over a side line. For both, non-offending team throws in and plays the ball.

Handball

A scoring area for handball is marked by chalk on a 3–4 metre radius. Only the goalkeeper may stand in this area.

2 versus 2, half-pitch, '3 lives' games

For the 2 versus 2, '3 lives' games, the class may choose amicably their favourite game to be played in half of the area.

Lesson Plan 8 • 30-45 minutes
April

Warm-up and Footwork Practices
4—6 minutes

1   Alternate jogging and sprinting. In your short sprints emphasise the straightening of the rear driving leg for power and the good lifting of the leading thigh for distance.

2   Teacher's-space tag. Can you cross from one side to the other of the area being 'guarded' by the teacher and four helpers with coloured bands, without being touched, to score a point? Helpers are changed over often and best scores for crossings are checked and praised.

Skills Practices: with short-tennis rackets and balls
8—12 minutes

Partner practices

1   One bowls gently underarm for partner to strike back for a catch by the bowler, using backhand and forehand strokes, standing side on to partner or where net would be. Change after 8 hits.

2   Racket each. Try to keep a rally going and return to readiness position, with both hands, after every stroke (illustrated), i.e. face partner with racket head held in front of body with its edge towards partner. Can you rally up to 8? Stand at least 12 metres apart, ideally with a line 'net' between you.

Group Practices and Small-sided Games
18—27 minutes

Short tennis

Teams of 4 or 5. Hit ball over net and run to back of own line. What is team's best score in a rally?

Rounders

4 or 5 a side, 3 catches. Batting team follow striker to score 1–4, depending on number of bases passed before fielders make 3 catches and shout 'Stop!'

2 v 2, side-to-side games

Choice of netball, floor-football, hockey, rugby-touch.

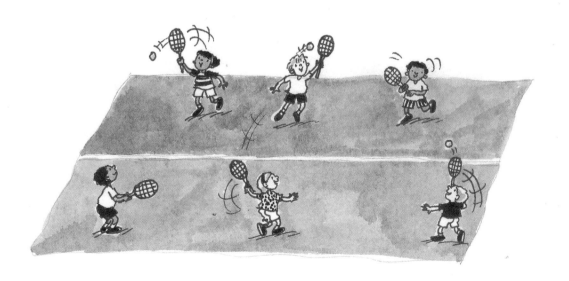

Games

Teaching notes and NC guidance
Development over 4–5 lessons

Lesson's main emphases:

a   The NC requirements to make judgements of performance and suggest ways to improve.

b   From now on, with the arrival of better weather, giving greater emphasis to reflection and evaluation during lessons, after demonstrations by individuals, pairs or groups. During the winter, such moments should have been few and very short to avoid loss of warmth. Even now, particularly in the 30 minute lesson, the teacher should warn the demonstrators that they will be performing to show a certain feature of the work, so that they are standing ready for an immediate start.

Take about 40 seconds to cover the following: 'Stop everyone! Watch how Thomas and Sarah are rallying well in short tennis. Tell me, after the demonstration, why they are being so successful and making long rallies', then the observation, the small sample of answers, and 'Thank you for the excellent demonstration and answers. Now continue and try to use some of the features that were praised.' At the start of each new set of lessons we should put the class 'in the picture' regarding the lesson's main aims and content. It seems a good idea, also, to put them in the picture regarding the value of the demonstrations, spoken reflection and evaluation. But it must not be allowed to monopolise the lesson, as is often the case.

Equipment: 30 short-tennis rackets and balls; 4 cones as bases in rounders; large balls; hockey sticks and balls; netball apparatus for choice of 2 versus 2 games across thirds of the netball court.

Group Practices and Small-sided Games

Short tennis

Short-tennis net is paint line on playground, low, long rope tied between netball posts, or long rope tied between chairs. A target circle of chalk on each side, about 5 metres from the net, helps the striker to aim at a point where the receiver is hoping the ball will come. Encourage 'Help your receiver by hitting to the forehand side.'

Rounders

In 3-catch-rounders the ball must be kept within the third of the netball court or long, wild hitting will ruin the game. The 3 catches must be made among 3 different players of the fielding side. Batting team's score is determined by number of cones passed by the whole team, with a maximum of 4, but teams might suggest another system. For example, the striker alone might be allowed to continue running to gain extra team points.

2 v 2, side-to-side games

A choice of four games for 2 versus 2 in a smallish rectangle. The two (or same) games chosen would each be played in half of the third used for this practice. The players would stay with their choice of game for one lesson, but would be allowed to change the following week, or the pairings could be changed from week to week for variety.

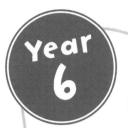

Year 6

Lesson Plan 9 • 30–45 minutes
May

Warm-up and Footwork Practices
4–6 minutes

1   Run and jump high and run and jump long over the lines on our playground. Find out which foot you push off with in a high jump and in a long jump. It's not always the same one.

2   Partner watches height of your standing high jump over a line or cane held by partner. Feet slightly apart, swing arms up, down behind, then spring up strongly from both feet. Pull knees up for maximum height.

Skills Practices: with small balls
8–12 minutes

Partner practices

1   At different distances throw and catch underarm and overarm. At what distance apart do you change from one to the other?

2   Across the netball court, practise bowling underarm or overarm to each other. Aim to make ball bounce a 'good length' (about 1 metre) in front of partner.

3   Backstop rolls ball for fielder to run, pick up and throw firmly just above wicket or cone height to the stationary wicketkeeper or backstop. Change over after 6 practices.

Invent a Skills Practice in 2s — 3–5 minutes

Invent a practice to develop throwing, catching, fielding, wicketkeeping. (For example, batter uses hand to strike ball at target line 'wicket', then runs to bowler's mark and back if he hits ball gently past fielders. Players decide on how batter can be 'out'.)

Group Practices and Small-sided Games
15–22 minutes

Stoolball

In 4s, half court, 2 groups. After five bowls all rotate around one position (batter, bowler, backstop, fielder). Batter runs to bowler's end to score a run.

Volleyball

2 v 2 over high rope 'net' between posts. Long rally volleying, both hands. 3 volleys each side. Groups can decide how to re-start after a rally.

Skipping rope each or long rope, team skipping

Quick, 1-beat action; 1 skip per rope turn. Slower, 2-beat action; 2 skips per turn. With long rope, work out best way to enter, start skipping, and leave it (illustrated).

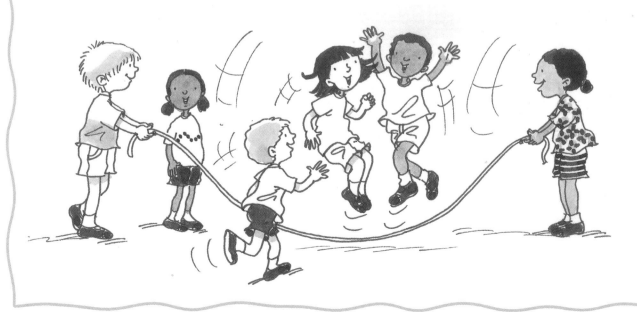

Games

Teaching notes and NC guidance
Development over 4–5 lessons

Lesson's main emphases:

a   The NC requirements to improve the skills of sending, receiving and striking the ball in net and striking/fielding games, and to plan, perform and reflect, for example on their own created games.

b   Recognising and valuing the variety that has always been a feature of these playground games lessons. There is variety in the lesson plan itself – warm-up, skills practices, invent a game or practice, and 3 varied games. Over the year as a whole there is good variety, with the change to net and striking/fielding games and athletic activities during the summer term. We want all our children to enjoy their Games lessons, to remember them with pleasure because they were interesting, challenging, exciting and varied, meaning that there was always at least some part of each lesson that they really enjoyed. Such enjoyment and good memories, while at school, are a main incentive to continuing to participate as adults in some forms of physical activity.

Equipment: 15 small balls; 1 set of stoolball apparatus; 1 long rope 'net' tied high between netball apparatus and 2 large balls for volleyball; 10 skipping ropes and 2 long skipping ropes.

Warm-up and Footwork Practices

1   Be aware of your take-off foot in high and long jumps. Use the scissor high jump, swinging non-jumping foot over an imaginary bar, and landing on it first. In long jumps, with a long straight leg reaching out in front of you, land gently on both feet.

2   The 2-foot take-off, after a long swing back of both arms and a preparatory knee bend, is an explosive spring up to land on both feet. Partner judges 'As high as my waist: Well done.'

Skills Practices: with small balls

The three practices – throwing and catching; bowling; fielding, then throwing to wicketkeeper – all lend themselves to continuous practice if teacher ensures that the distances apart are sensible and not too wide.

Group Practices and Small-sided Games

Stoolball

Stoolball is a cross between rounders and cricket. The bowl to batter is like rounders and the running between the posts is like cricket. Ways to be 'out' are like cricket, and the class can agree one main rule and suggest ways to be 'out' to keep all fielders on their toes.

Volleyball

In volleyball, aim to volley high enough each time to lift ball above partner for a good return volley. It is co-operative, trying for a long rally together. With beginners, one bounce on the ground might be allowed, to be followed by striking the ball above own or another's head for the next volley.

Skipping rope each or long rope, team skipping

In long rope, team skipping, 'Can 2 or 3 of you come in to, then leave the rope, after skipping together as a group?'

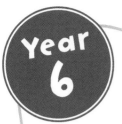

Year 6

Lesson Plan 10 • 30-45 minutes
June

Warm-up and Footwork Practices
4—6 minutes

1 The outside measurement of the netball court is approximately 90 metres. Run at a comfortable speed for a minute and let me see how many circuits and metres you can do, compared with your own estimate.

2 2s, standing broad jump from a side line. Your partner will mark your distance. Try 3 jumps and use (a) toes turned in slightly at start, (b) a strong backward, then forward arm swing and (c) a long, low stretch out of body in flight.

Skills Practices: with large balls
8—12 minutes

Group of 3 players:

1 Volley pass and follow your pass.

2 2 balls on move. Can you pressurise middle person?

3 If you have a wall, can you keep ball going, volleying to rebound to yourself?

Group Practices and Small-sided Games
18—27 minutes

Volleyball or Newcombe

2 a side at high 'net' rope between netball posts. In Newcombe, receiver may catch and hold ball for a moment before 2-hand return over net. Ball may be interpassed on same side 3 times before being sent over net (illustrated). No 1-handed play allowed.

Circular-cricket

1 bowler, 2 batters, 1 wicketkeeper, 4 fielders. Rotate to new position every 5 or 6 balls.

2 v 2 over line 'net', hand-tennis, short tennis or quoits

Serve from own rear line. Play 4-point game and then change sides. Encourage players to communicate with partners to cover front and rear of own court and to decide who will return a ball between them. Winning or losing couples can compete.

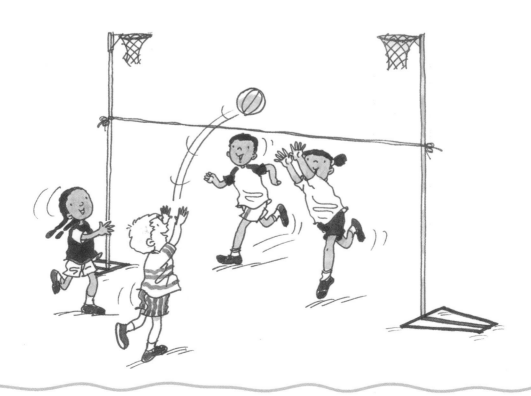

Games

Teaching notes and NC guidance
Development over 4–5 lessons

Lesson's main emphases:

a The NC requirements to improve the skills of sending and receiving a ball in net and striking/fielding games, and to practise, adapt, improve and repeat longer and increasingly complex sequences of movement.

b A stepping back by the teacher, as the class come to the end of Key Stage 2 and primary school, to observe and reflect on:

1 Is there an atmosphere of quiet but busy, purposeful activity with all physically and whole-heartedly active, and demonstrating a pleasing level of skilfulness and versatility?

2 Is there an impression of independence and understanding with the class able to organise itself in a co-operative way, without the teacher always needing to step in to get something started?

3 Is there an impression of good sporting behaviour and making allowances for teammates of different (lesser) abilities? Are all children given their turn and helped to take part?

4 Is everything that is happening good, safe practice? Are the class sensibly dressed, having changed for the lesson, and without jewellery? Is there a total lack of any form of anti-social, selfish or dangerous behaviour?

5 Is there an obvious impression of children at play, thoroughly enjoying themselves and having great fun together?

Equipment: 10 large balls; 1 set of Kwik cricket; 10 short-tennis rackets and 3 balls; quoits as alternative choice for 2 versus 2 games.

Skills Practices: with large balls

Volleying is difficult and if some children are finding it impossible to do well, let them have one bounce in between volleys. After the bounce, the ball can be played up to a partner with a 'dig' with front of forearms. Hands are clasped, arms are low and straight with front of forearms used to hit the ball up with a long, smooth swing, helped by a stretching of the knees.

Group Practices and Small-sided Games

Volleyball or Newcombe

If the skill level is low, play Newcombe, where you may hold ball momentarily on fingertips, before bending and stretching the arms to send it on its way. If skill level is average, they can try, co-operatively, to make a long rally. If skill level is very good, they can play 2 versus 2 competitively.

Circular-cricket

If there are 2 netball courts, one can be used for the circular-cricket so that a 20-metre wicket can be used and a bigger playing area.

2 v 2 over line 'net', hand-tennis, short tennis or quoits

Over the low 'net', playing a competitive 2 versus 2 game, their ability level should help decide which game they will play – the easiest quoits, the fairly easy hand-tennis, or the more difficult short tennis with rackets.

Lesson Plan 11 • 30–45 minutes
July

Warm-up and Footwork Practices
4–5 minutes

1 Run anti-clockwise around netball court, then jog end third, sprint middle third, jog end third. Turn and repeat. Count the number of foot strikes needed to take you across the middle third and try to reduce this number by better knee lift and stronger rear leg action.

2 2s, side line sprint relay. Stand side by side down centre of court. Race on signal to touch nearer side line with foot; turn and race back to touch partner's hand. Teacher calls 'make six hand touches. Go!'

Skills Practices: with short-tennis rackets and balls
6–10 minutes

Partner practices

1 One bowls underarm to batting partner about 4 metres away, who strikes it back, forehand, to bowler. Change over after 8 practices. Which couple can make the most catches before dropping one?

2 Have a competition with your partner, alternating striking ball up a short distance using forehand and backhand grips, i.e. palm facing up, then knuckles facing up.

Group Practices and Small-sided Games
20–30 minutes

Short tennis

2 v 2. Drop on end line, serve with a forehand hit. Change sides after a 4-point game. Ask teams to suggest fair ways to serve to start and restart games, for example by drop and hit from behind own line to person diagonally opposite.

Tip-and-run cricket

4 or 5 a side. Challenge cricketers to agree a way to keep game moving so that no outstanding batter keeps 1 team at wicket, for example batters help to field before and after being 'in' (illustrated).

Volleyball

4 a side over high rope 'net' between netball posts. Allow 3 volleys on each side of net. Score while serving. Team rotates around after a loss of service. Challenge volleyers to agree a 'friendly' rule to help game keep moving, for example one bounce allowed on each side.

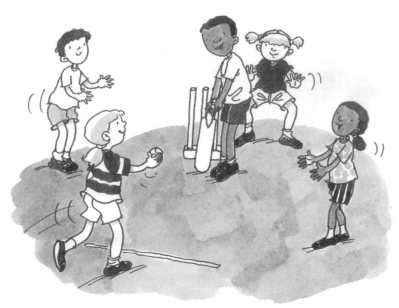

Games

Teaching notes and NC guidance
Development over 4–5 lessons

Lesson's main emphases:

a The Performing. Are skilfulness and ability evident in the neat, efficient, controlled, poised and adaptable way the skills are being used? Are the children versatile and successful performers?

b The Planning. Are their performances well organised, clearly focused and successful because they are 'seeing' ahead to guide them to be in the right place to do the right action, at the right time?

c The Reflecting/Evaluating. Following a performance, can they demonstrate that they are careful, accurate observers who can recognise main features; express pleasure about certain aspects; identify contrasting actions; and make good judgements as they suggest areas for improvement, at all times using language that is appropriate?

Equipment: 30 short-tennis rackets and balls; 1 Kwik cricket set; high rope 'net' tied between netball posts and 2 large balls for volleyball; low, long rope 'net' between chairs for tennis.

Warm-up and Footwork Practices

1 A better knee-lift action and longer stride takes you to the line quicker if rhythm of running stays the same.

2 The relay can be speeded up by runner jumping to turn and face partner at line; by partner crouching at start for a quicker take off; by both using short, rapid strides.

Skills Practices: with short-tennis rackets and balls

Partner practices

1 The signal for the bowler to serve ball to batter is the batter taking racket from ready position in both hands back to start of forehand hit position, body turned side on to bowler. Ball is aimed to bounce up on forehand side between chest and shoulder.

2 Each has a ball and counts own score, hitting ball straight up and down, with racket face turning each time.

Group Practices and Small-sided Games

Short tennis

In short tennis, the non-server can stand at the 'net' to cover the return of service, as a simple tactic.

Tip-and-run cricket

Play tip-and-run cricket on a second netball court if there is one, with the outside lines the ball's limit.

Volleyball

If a one bounce suggestion is made, it helps to remind the players to 'dig' the ball up after the bounce if it is too low to volley. The dig would be extra to the three volleys allowed to each team before ball must be played over the net.